WHAT ARE YOU WAITING FOR?

FROM THE COUCH TO RUNNING THE SEVEN CONTINENTS

Published in Australia by Sid Harta Books & Print Pty Ltd,
ABN: 34632585293
23 Stirling Crescent, Glen Waverley, Victoria 3150 Australia
Telephone: +61 3 9560 9920, Facsimile: +61 3 9545 1742
E-mail: author@sidharta.com.au

First published in Australia 2021
This edition published 2021
Copyright © Michael le Page 2021
Cover design, typesetting: WorkingType (www.workingtype.com.au)

Le Page, Michael
What Are You Waiting For?
ISBN: 978-1-925707-47-2
pp336

WHAT ARE YOU WAITING FOR?

FROM THE COUCH TO RUNNING THE SEVEN CONTINENTS

MICHAEL LE PAGE

To Maria, my wife, my best friend, my running partner, my travelling companion, my accountant, and my advisor.

To Jewel, our friend, marathon partner, seven continent marathoner, and Marathon des Sables competitor.

To Barbara Ivusic for the editing, Alaine Neilson for the proofreading of the text and Luke Harris of WorkingType Design for the typesetting and cover design.

Table of Contents

Preface

People regularly approach my wife Maria and me and say that they've heard we had run a marathon in Antarctica or along the Great Wall of China or in the Valley of the Queens in Egypt or a marathon on all seven continents. We try to explain the experience, but they often respond that we should write the story down, so it's not lost.

Maria and I are based in Perth, Australia. We are not professional athletes, but working parents of four and have taken our passion for running to the point where it led us to run marathons and ultramarathons around the world. Of the 7.8 billion people in the world, 818 have run a marathon on each continent and joined the seven-continent club. We are two of them. It started as a casual jog, then turned into a five-kilometre run, and then progressed to crossing the finish line of the most famous marathon of them all. If you are not a runner, we hope this will encourage you to put on your shoes, step outside, enjoy the fresh air and go for a run. If you are a runner, we hope it will encourage you to take the next step and set some exciting running goals. As our friend Jewel wrote 'Go ahead, change your life.' Here is our story.

Chapter 1

Barefoot in the frost

What's wrong? 'He's very sick', someone whispered. 'Move along, get dressed and have some breakfast,' said the lady of the house. She was a five-foot-tall, pale, slim, Irish lady who had immigrated to Australia at eighteen years of age to work as a children's nurse in Sydney. She had pale green eyes and auburn hair which was starting to be streaked with glimpses of grey as she moved into her late thirties. She was a loving but determined lady who adored her husband, but it looked like he was sick now, very sick indeed.

She was our mother, and our dad was the one who was sick in bed and couldn't get up. 'Severe chest pain' were the words that filtered through to us as we crowded around the breakfast table eating Kellogg's cereal and getting ready for school. He was forty-three years old, too young to be that sick. He was short but broad at the shoulders and was in his youth a pugilist. His fame in the ring was to win all his bouts except when his father came to see him fight. Unfortunately for him, his father only came once, and it was in the final of the year's championship. He had one green eye and one which was green tinged with yellow from an accident in his youth when he was struck in the eye with something which made him blind in one eye. I never found out for sure what caused the blindness. One rumour was a slingshot accident, another was a tennis ball accident. It was a topic that I never broached with him and I'm not sure why. It just never came up. I do regret that, though. My older brother said it was an accident with a cricket ball.

The doctor was called for a house visit as Dad was too sick to travel, and it was common in those days for the doctor to visit. Nowadays, an ambulance would be called, and he would go to the emergency ward at the hospital. The doctor was Dr Stuart, our family doctor. Then, most people had a family doctor who knew them, took the time to understand all the family's medical issues and visit the home when required regardless of the time of day or night for an emergency. Time has moved on. Medical doctors now have great computer systems to record data, look for trends and allow other doctors to fill in when needed. We also knew his father who was Dr Merv. Apparently studying medicine was a family trait as Dr Stuart's son also became a doctor.

Dr Stuart's wife was ahead of her time and was known for planting trees in the parks around our neighbourhood.

She did it at her own expense and on her own time as she believed trees were very important, that we should treasure our flora and not be clearing land unnecessarily. She aimed to foster a caring nature in the community for the environment. Yes, it was the 1960s and she was well ahead of her time. Her trees still flourish today long after she died. People now just take it for granted the wonderful groves of native trees that flourish in that neighbourhood.

Dr Stuart duly arrived in his British-racing-green MG sports car. It always amazed me, that car. It was small, convertible, and represented to me a sense of being carefree with the wind gently caressing the face as he drove along with the roof down. Since then I have associated a convertible with independence and freedom. I'm not sure how I made that connection. The attraction for small convertibles has followed me all through life after seeing Dr Stuart arrive that day and on subsequent visits to our home. I have since owned a few convertibles. My first was a white 1964 Rootes Group Series IV Sunbeam Alpine and I still have a two-seat convertible now.

Dr Stuart was tall, lean, caring and walked leaning forward like he was in a hurry. Maybe he was. He appeared old to me. At my eleven years, someone being old was subjective, but he was probably around only forty years old then. He came in carrying his small bag of doctors' things which were a mystery to us kids watching his arrival through the upstairs window. We imagined lots of hypodermic needles, bottles of medicine and certainly a stethoscope in there too.

Thirty minutes later Dr Stuart duly departed, and our mother said, 'Dad is okay. He had his vitals checked and just needs some rest for the day and to take some aspirin.' That seemed simple enough.

Over the next few days Dad seemed to get better and I remember him saying, 'Dr Stuart thought that the chest pain was a warning and that I need to exercise a lot more, especially do some vigorous exercise to get fitter, stronger and leaner.' My dad was not prone to vigorous exercise or team sports in recent years. He was a spectator rather than a participant in active sports. He studied to be a scientist, worked in an office and a laboratory while his pastimes were playing lawn bowls and making and flying remote controlled model aeroplanes. During vacations, he would go beach fishing where he would stand for hours watching the sea playing cat and mouse with the fish. According to the doctor, at forty-three years old, Dad needed to do more than rolling a ball down a patch of lawn and standing around flying model aeroplanes or fishing. I guess the forty cigarettes a day didn't help his cause either.

Dr Stuart talked to him about a thing called jogging which was becoming popular. It started where athletes such as boxers or track-and-field athletes ran several kilometres each day as part of improving their fitness and conditioning. Apparently in New Zealand during the 1960s, the word 'jogging' was promoted by the coach Arthur Lydiard, who is credited with making jogging popular. It was also documented in a sports page article in *The New Zealand Herald* in February 1962. It told of a group of former athletes and fitness enthusiasts who would meet regularly to run to get and stay fit. In the article the newspaper suggested the words 'Joggers' Club' which is thought to be the first use of the noun jogger. The University of Oregon, USA, track coach Bill Bowerman, started a joggers' club in early 1963. He published the book *Jogging* in 1966. Jogging then was a form of running at a slow constant pace with the aim to increase physical fitness. It was less stressful than running and better than walking with the aim to maintain a constant pace for longer periods of time to increase aerobic fitness.

So, jogging came into our household in 1969. My father thought it was a good idea to do this and as such he also thought three of his four sons should accompany him every day at 5.30 am for a jog. The fourth son was too young at the time and he was pleased with the opportunity to not be up at 5.30 every morning. For my brothers and me, a 5.30 start was much earlier than we were used to, but we went along with Dad's enthusiasm. This would be my first introduction to jogging.

It was April 1969 and summer was moving into autumn. The concept of jogging for my dad was to briefly read the headlines of the local newspaper which was delivered to the front door of our home early each morning, then take off at a nice steady slow pace. It was somewhat less than slow running but faster that walking. He would head for the nearest park which for us was Limestone Park about 800 metres away. In the park was a cricket ground which was very green, and the perimeter was lined with a picturesque white picket fence. In the middle of the ground roughly aligned north to south was a rectangular clay strip covered with short grass. It was called the pitch on which the game of cricket was centred. The pitch was 20 metres long and made of a special black high clay soil as this helps the cricket pitch from forming cracks. The logic behind the north–south alignment is like tennis so that the sun would not be in the eyes of the players in the early morning or late afternoon. In Australia, grounds like this had multiple uses so here it was a cricket oval in summer and an Australian Rules football oval in winter. We would do four circuits of this ground which was about 600 metres around and head back home.

The last 50 metres of the jog involved a fast run to the end. It was, in his way, a nice way to finish the run. The total jog each morning was 4 kilometres or 2.5 miles. After that, my dad would do a few sit-ups, feel fitter, more energised, happy with himself and ready for the day. I did too.

For my brothers and me, a slow jog around the local park was great as we could spend some extra time with our dad who always seemed to be super busy. However, we both trained for football twice a week, played a football game once a week and on most other days played football in the park with our friends, so the jog was slow and 5.30 in the morning was early. We did enjoy the run and it was wonderful in the park in the early morning with the sun starting to rise and the masked lapwing plovers swooping about. They're a large, common native bird which spends most of its time on the ground searching for food such as insects and worms. The birds nest on the ground in the reeds near a swampy area of the park and they would swoop any person or dog that came within their territory, a natural behaviour to protect their eggs and young. Swooping birds were to visit my life again in the future on a different, much colder continent.

Over time our dad got fitter but not faster, and I think my brothers and I got fitter as well. We found playing football games easier and races at school as well, but perhaps more importantly, it was nice to spend that time with our dad. He was a gregarious, very intelligent man who liked academic pursuits but was not philosophical. Along the way he would chat about what was happening in the world or at work and he would occasionally remind us to be respectful and honest and to work and study hard as these values were important to him. The world he spoke of seemed a faraway place for us from our own community and school. Every now and then he would also remind us to own up to and learn from our mistakes. Values were not necessarily taught in a formal way, but you absorbed them from your parents, family, school, and community life.

As autumn drifted into winter, the air in the mornings became colder and frost started to appear occasionally on our morning run. As we lived in a subtropical climate, much like parts of Florida in the US, it was pleasant all year around but hot in summer and cool enough in winter for frost, but never cold enough for snow. When the temperature dipped, Limestone Park would be covered in white frosting early in the morning.

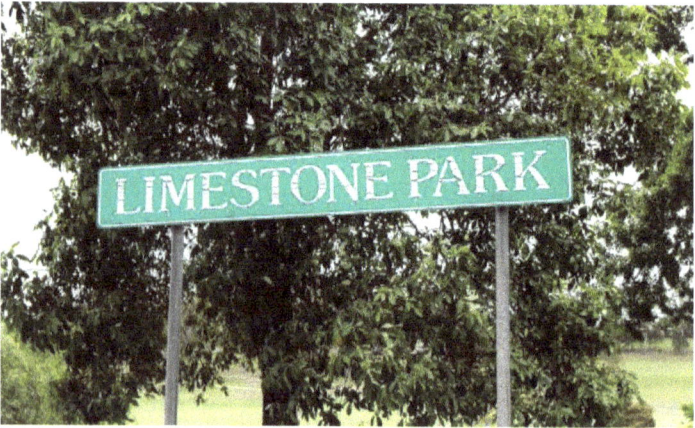

Limestone Park, Ipswich, Australia (Originally Ipswich was called 'The Limestone Hills' or 'Limestone' as lime was quarried there)

At home there was no central heating or cooling and we only required an extra blanket or two on the bed at night and a jumper for school in winter. Shorts and long socks were the norm all year around at school. In fact, I didn't own a pair of long pants until I was thirteen and in high school. I still recall the old grey or black ex-army blankets we used in winter on the beds.

So, when we went jogging with our dad in winter, we realised that bare foot running in winter with a frost covering the ground was not ideal. We could deal with the dirt, the odd pebble, crossing the rough bitumen road and thorns on the ground during the rest of the year but frost was a bit too much. At the end of one morning run, I looked down at my feet and they were tinged in blue. I was cold and my feet felt frozen. My dad noticed as well, and he suggested that my brothers and I should get some shoes for running and a jogging sweatshirt to keep warm.

In 1969 running shoes designed for joggers really didn't exist in Australia. The Adidas Rome running shoe was manufactured in leather from 1958 ahead of the Rome Olympics but was not a mainstream low-cost running shoe at the time. Their competitor's Pumas running shoes were also not commonly available either. The only available shoes for us and our budget were the sandshoe or sneaker which had a white canvas upper and a rubber sole with a lace-up to secure the shoe. It was used for some sports like tennis and athletics. The other shoe was a gym boot which was a high ankle lace up shoe much like a modern Converse branded shoe. We never had a gym to go to, so we never owned any gym boots. Oddly enough, Converse gym shoes were the most famous and popular basketball shoes until Nike introduced the Air Jordan basketball shoe. The sandshoes or sneakers as they were sometimes called had a simple style and an advanced style. The advanced style was the more expensive Dunlop Volley which was marketed as a tennis shoe. Tennis stars like Australia's Rod Laver and Margaret Court reportedly wore the Dunlop Volley tennis shoe. The word 'Volley' came from the tennis shot of the same name. For our running at the time the only real choice was the lower cost, basic sandshoe.

There was another member of the family who really took up this jogging with enormous enthusiasm. That was the Labrador dog named Hannibal. He was not our dog but belonged to the family who lived down the road. He adopted us and, on most days, he stayed at our house and often slept there as well. At that time, where we lived, we rarely locked up the house and Hannibal would roam in and out day or night as the back door was always ajar or fully open. I had never heard of a robbery or house break-in. I grew up not having a house key or even knowing where to find one.

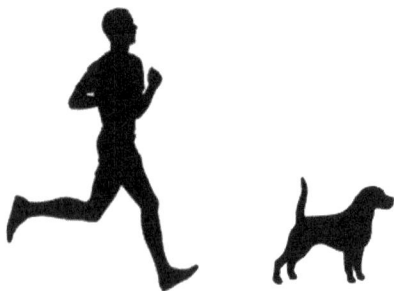

At 5.30 am, by means of a dog alarm clock, Hannibal would go into my parents' room, sit by my father's side

and start whining for him to wake up and go jogging. Like most dogs he would run twice as far as us chasing the plovers, smelling trees, running ahead and back to us and so on. Hannibal was by far the most fanatical jogger in the family. And so began my love for running. I found I enjoyed the fresh air, the views, the exertion, and the feeling of wellness after a run in nature. Perhaps it was a bit of escapism as well to get away from everything and just run.

By the time I reached high school a year later, my running had improved. The fastest runners in my grade were soon coming second to me in longer races and I was always selected for the top football team and sometimes for the football team above my grade as well as the regional teams. Perhaps jogging daily was producing results. I recall one cross country race for the high school. It was a handicap race with the younger runners starting off first and the older Year 12 students starting off last. The race was five kilometres of trails and I ran in first from the whole school. My younger brother, Mark, was also very successful in those cross-country races throughout high school and my older brother, Arthur, evolved into a very capable 1500-metre runner. There were inter-school competitions throughout my high school years with some wins and some losses but the love of running from those humble beginnings with my dad jogging around the park in bare feet stayed with me for life. It was not an all- encompassing passion for running as some people have but a lifelong enjoyable thing to do. I still have an image in my mind of my dad jogging around Limestone Park in the winter mornings shuffling along, faster than a walk and slower than a slow run.

'To keep the body in good health is a duty. Otherwise we shall not be able to keep our mind strong and clear.'
— Buddha

Chapter 2

'On on' in the rainforest

'**S**elamat pagi, selamat sore, selamat siang, selamat malam, apa kabah, baik baik saja' he repeated. ('Good morning. Good afternoon. Good evening. How are you? Fine, fine.'). My Indonesian teacher, Pak Walas, patiently took me for a lesson each Tuesday afternoon so I could learn the language Bahasa, the common language across Indonesia. My wife Maria and I had moved there for work as I got a position as an industrial chemist in my mid-twenties. It was the beginning of a reinvigorated running journey for me, the start of a running journey for my wife Maria, and an amazing period of personal development for both of us.

Indonesia is a country just to the north of Australia between the Indian and Pacific Oceans and south of Singapore and Malaysia. Many people, especially Australians, know it, as the island of Bali is a common and wonderful tropical holiday destination. Indonesia is the world's largest island country with more than seventeen thousand islands and an area of 1.9 million square kilometres or approximately 735 000 square miles. It is the fourteenth largest country by land area with over 260 million people. This makes it the world's fourth most populous country as well as the most populous Muslim-majority country. Java, the world's most populous island, is home to more than half of the country's population and the country's capital, Jakarta, is the second most populous urban area in the world behind Tokyo and ahead of Manila.

The country is along the equator and the climate tends to be relatively even all year round. It has two seasons which are a wet season and a dry season so there are no extremes of summer or winter. For most of Indonesia, the dry season falls between May and October with the wet season between November and April. The climate is tropical with tropical rainforests found in every large island of Indonesia.

In Indonesia there are more than 700 languages. It has the reputation as the second most linguistically diverse nation in the world. There is, however, a national language which is referred to as Bahasa Indonesia and is a standardised form of the Malaysian language. Javanese is the largest language by the number of native speakers.

So, for us, two adult Australians with two very young children, the relocation to the city of Bandung, which is the fourth most populous city in Indonesia, was a very adventurous change. The greater urban area holds over 8.5 million people and it is situated up in the mountains 140 kilometres or 87 miles from Jakarta on the island of Java. We moved from an Australian town with 70 000 people who were almost all white, taller, heavier, Anglo-Saxon origin, English-speaking, Christian and relatively insular. The Indonesians on the other hand were mainly brown, short, thin, light in weight, Asian, Indonesian-speaking, Muslims and relatively insular too. But they were very friendly and welcoming. We never felt intimated or afraid but were cautious with food and water because we didn't want to get sick. I had never heard of a Muslim nor knew anything about the country except I read a book by the Australian novelist Christopher John Koch called *The Year of Living Dangerously* which was about the dramatic overthrow of the first president of Indonesia, Sukarno, to the new president Suharto in 1967. A novel centred around a love story is not a good way to learn about a country nor the things you may encounter.

I'm five-foot-nine-inches (175 cm) and weighed at the time 75 kilograms or 165 pounds. Thirty-five years later I'm still the same weight but may have shrunk in height over time. In the US, my height is the average height for a male, but the average weight is 198 pounds with a waist size of 40 inches, which is 33 pounds heavier than me. My waist is 30 inches. So, in the US I would be described as average height and lean. In Indonesia, however, I was considered very tall, much taller than almost everyone else and much heavier, so much so that I wasn't able to buy any shoes as my feet were too big, or shirts as my chest was too large or jeans as my waist was too big. I'm also white-skinned and had fair hair and green eyes, so I stood out significantly as did Maria and our two children. Maria is dark-haired, tall, and lean as well. You would call her, even at over sixty now, athletic in build. She too had trouble buying clothes and shoes. I recall taking the family to the zoo one day to see the animals and the biggest crowd there was around us and our two, fair-haired, white infant boys.

I did come away from Indonesia being far more experienced in many things. I learned a lot in my work, especially on how to deal with customers in a different country and culture. I learned how to eat in an environment where the hygiene standards were much lower than I was used to. I only drank water that had been boiled for twenty minutes and always cleaned the top of a drink bottle after the cap was prised off. Bottled water was not available then as it is now. I also only ate fruit and vegetables that we peeled, plus, at the time I did not consume any dairy products. This was combined with regular washing of the hands, never using water to brush our teeth, and keeping our mouths closed when showering. These became our standard procedures and I still adhere to this when I travel to places where I have concerns with food hygiene and water purity. Over the entire time we lived in Indonesia we never got sick and in all our travels around the world since we never gotten sick as well. I learned a lot of other things as well. I became much more tolerant, more tolerant of our differences like race and religion, and more understanding of the real meaning of poverty and corruption. Because I needed to learn another language quickly and to understand a different culture, I became much more tolerant and respectful of people who move to a new country and need to learn a whole other language. I was lucky to have just joined a group of people who really enjoyed working internationally and were not afraid to travel, to do business in different countries or to live in different places. We were inspired by both the experience and the people with whom I worked plus the many expatriates we met along the journey.

So how did we end up in Indonesia? As time passed, I went to university, gained an applied science degree majoring in chemistry, and moved away from home to start my first full time job in northern Queensland, Australia at a country town called Collinsville. My university days had required me to commute about two hours each way from home to university and back involving a walk to the train station, an hour's train ride then another walk to the university. Although sometimes I was driven to the train station in the morning, I walked home in the evening. Consequently, my football training stopped as study was the ticket to future opportunities. Running also stopped but each weekend I would still go for the occasional long run to satisfy my love of the run. Dad still went jogging on most mornings. It was his ritual and when he died years later it was not from a heart attack or a cardiovascular problem but from cancer, so his morning jog had most probably prolonged his life, kept him mentally sharp and provided a much-improved quality of life for him.

We applied for a job in Indonesia after moving several times up and down the east coast of Australia. It seemed like a good opportunity at the time and would provide an adventure for us all as well as significant work experience. I read that the poet William Wordsworth once said, 'Poetry is the spontaneous overflow of powerful feelings: it takes its origin from emotion recollected in tranquillity'. Living in Indonesia at that time was like that, as when I look back, I ignore all the ups and downs of life there and only reflect on it as a great adventure.

Yet, in Indonesia there were many challenges. We were robbed in daylight at our house by an intruder armed with a large knife who terrorised Maria and the children while I was at work. Fortunately, after he took what money and jewellery we had, he left the house on his own accord. Subsequently, we hired 24-hour guards at the house to avoid being robbed again. We also couldn't drink the water. Malaria was rife in parts of the country and the malaria medication, Chloroquine, induced depression in us. You also needed to be very careful with what and where to eat to avoid hepatitis, food poisoning, diarrhoea, and intestinal worms. Infant mortality was ten per cent in the country and corruption was present, but with the benefit of hindsight and recollection in tranquillity many years later, life in Indonesia was a wonderful, event- filled adventure. It made our family stronger, more resilient, and more adventurous.

On the upside, when we moved to Indonesia, we had several house staff to help us with the normal chores of cleaning, cooking, washing clothes, child minding and gardening. It was normal in Indonesia to provide work for people as labour was plentiful and relatively inexpensive plus it provided jobs and income for people. The house staff were generally good and easy to have around the house. This provided my wife and I time to be away from the children, so we joined a running club.

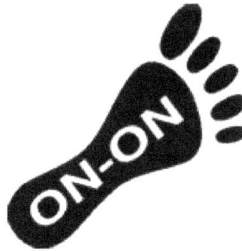

Now, at that time the Bandung Hash House Harriers (HHH) were reportedly the biggest single HHH club in the world. It was so big in fact that we split the club into two groups because we had trouble finding places to run which had adequate space to park cars. There was and still is in 2020 Bandung HHH 1 which runs on Monday and Bandung HHH 2 which runs on Friday. The Hash House

Harriers is a group of non-competitive running clubs which started in Malaysia and has grown worldwide. It's a mixture of athleticism, hard work, and socialising plus a refreshing break from the six-day-a-week work routine. According to folklore, it began in Kuala Lumpur, Malaysia, in 1938, when a group of British men started a running group. They named the group after their meeting place, the Selangor Club, aka the 'Hash House'. Hash House Harrier runs were modelled on the traditional British public school paper chase.

The HHH met each Monday evening to chase a trail of small pieces of paper over the rainforests surrounding the region. An earlier run was set up for those who wanted a shorter run, and a longer run was for those semi-serious and serious runners. The long runs were typically 8–10 kilometres or 5–6 miles. The trails were set by different people each week and were full of false trails, sudden stops requiring backtracking, long runs up and down long mountain paths, runs through kampungs (villages), through beautiful rainforests and always ending up back at the start to have a celebration with a few drinks and lots of songs. During the HHH run when someone was leading the chase of the small pieces of paper in the rain forest they called *'on on'* to let everyone else know that they had found the trail and people could recommence running.

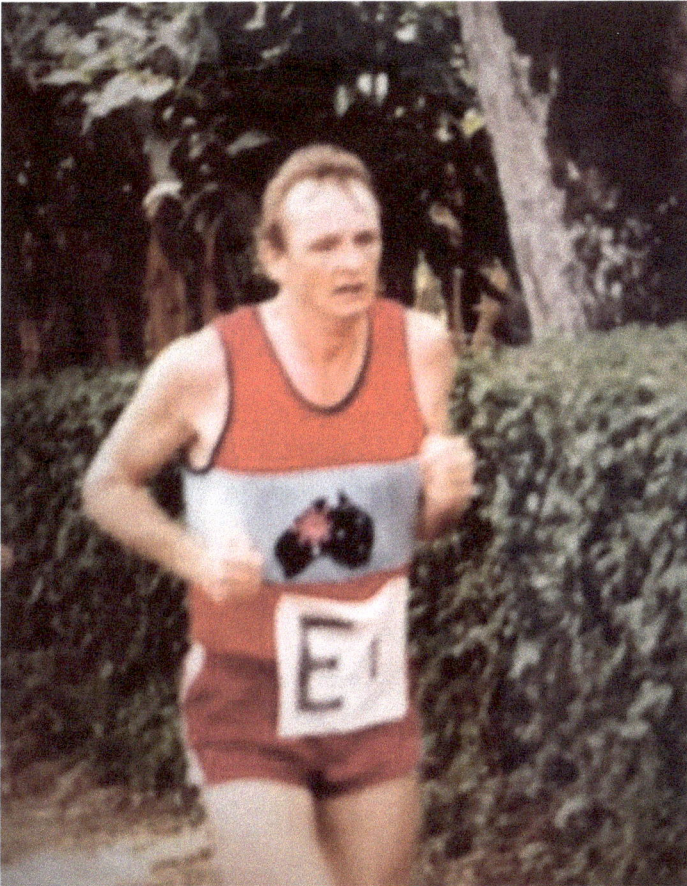

Michael — running in Indonesia

It was here we met many new friends, mainly expatriates from all over the world, who came together each Monday to run, catch up, have fun with a few songs and a few beers but just as importantly to provide friendship and support to each other when in sickness or in good health. It was here where I met some good runners, and we would go on extra runs during the week as that is what runners do. I was still playing football and had upgraded my shoes to what would now be called a trail shoe with small dimples on the sole for extra traction on country trails. As we ran along, the runners talked about if they were wearing their ripple shoes that day or some other shoe. This was all new to me.

It was here that Maria had, for the first time in her life, the opportunity to be in a running environment and run with good runners, let alone a running club. It was here that she blossomed into a wonderful runner who not only enjoyed the open spaces, and had great endurance but learned to run fast. She was a natural running talent and quickly became one of the best two runners not just in the club but within the expatriate community. With it she developed a real long-lasting passion for running. However, the time came for us to move back from Indonesia and back to normality. With it came a loss of household staff and back came the normal workload that comes with a growing family. Unfortunately, running had to take a back seat to the other priorities in life.

'Life brings tears, smiles and memories: the tears
dry, the smile fades, but the memories live on forever.'
— Anonymous

Chapter 3

A message from Steve

Sometimes certain events in life act as an unexpected immediate catalyst for long-lasting change like my dad with his health incident. For me, one day in 2004 I received a message from my friend Steve and many years later, because of acting on that message, I found myself standing on the foredeck of a ship heading to Antarctica. I was crossing from Ushuaia at the southern tip of Argentina, past the Wollaston Islands, past Cape Horn across the Drake Passage where the Atlantic and Pacific Oceans meet.

This is one of the most hazardous, rarely predictable shipping routes in the world as the waters around Cape Horn are dangerous due to strong winds, large waves, strong currents, and icebergs. The warm waters from the north and cold waters from the south collide to form strong eddies and when combined with other elements can sometimes create powerful storms. Fortunately, it was calm, and I really enjoyed the beautiful early morning in this part of the world as the sun started to rise over the blue green ocean. I woke early and, as the cabins on the vessel were small, I quietly left my room and started to walk around the deck. Most of the passengers were asleep but there was another person at the bow of the vessel, and he was standing by the railing looking out to sea.

We started talking. He was South African and was on board with his family of adult children plus his wife taking the trip. They were all runners except him. His real passion was birdwatching and he had expensive looking binoculars hanging around his neck with a well-used brown binocular case in his right hand. He loved birding or birdwatching he told me. It was his main recreational activity and the key reason he wanted to travel to Antarctica. He showed me some examples of the birds skimming the open sea in front of us. They were beautiful and graceful. Several species of Albatross passed by with their large wingspan as we spoke, and he pointed out a few Cape petrels with their distinctive black head and neck and white underbelly.

He said, 'The large white bird is the wandering albatross, is native to this area and has the largest wingspan of any bird in the world at around three metres.' Sadly, one albatross had become tangled overnight in the wire ropes stretching from the deck up to one of the masts and had broken its wing. The crew had called the marine biologist who was on board and she decided that the bird was not able to be treated. It was sadly lifted off the deck and let go overboard. We watched as it forlornly sat on the surface waiting its fate as the water trailed behind the vessel.

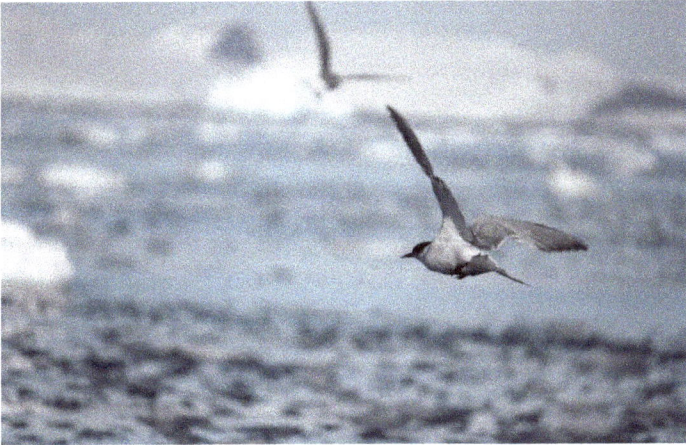

Birds in Antarctica

He spoke of his wife, of whom you could see he was immensely proud, and of her amazing achievements with an awe-inspiring story. Ten years ago, his family were sitting, watching on television the famous, long road race in South Africa called the Comrades Ultramarathon. It is the world's largest and oldest ultramarathon race and is labelled 'the ultimate human race'. The 89 kilometre or 55.6 mile gruelling road race is held each year from Durban to Pietermaritzburg in the province of KwaZulu-Natal and it must be completed within twelve hours. It changes direction each year with it starting in Durban one year and ending in Durban the following year.

Geography-wise this meant an uphill race one year and downhill the next. His wife said at the time while watching the race on the television, almost to herself, that she could do the Comrades Marathon. Her children looked at their mum, a middle-aged, unfit, non- runner, and laughed. Well that moment had an immediate impact on her and the next day she went out and bought some shoes and running clothes and started her running journey. Her runs were tentative and short at first, but her determination started to show through. She got fitter, leaner and her run distances longer. The family started to sit up and take notice that Mum was changing. A serious runner was emerging. They still thought that she would simply keep the running as a hobby for a while then it would fade away like a fad.

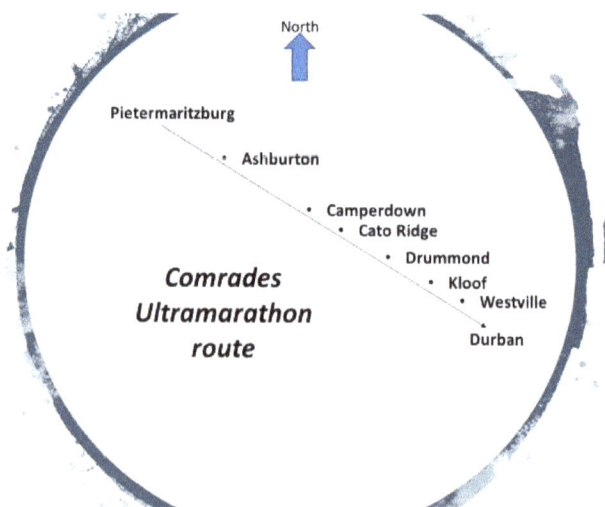

North

Pietermaritzburg

Ashburton

Camperdown
Cato Ridge
Drummond
Kloof
Westville
Durban

Comrades Ultramarathon route

Comrades Ultramarathon route

Her next step much to everyone's surprise was to register and run some races. Sure enough in time she competed the qualifying standard marathon of 42.2 kilometres (26.2 miles) within the cut-off time of five hours and then the Comrades 89-kilometre marathon the same year and each of the ten years since earning her the coveted green number as a finisher of ten Comrades races. Not only did it motivate each of her children to start running, now she and they were on their way to run a marathon in the bitterly cold, harsh, most isolated continent of Antarctica.

My wife also had a similar catalyst. One year I had run a 12-kilometre road race called City to Surf in my hometown. It is a very popular race involving 40 000 people starting from the centre of the city and ending at the beach near our house. It was convenient as I could walk home at the end of the race. My football days had ended as I was travelling a lot doing business in Asia. This is what I dreamt of doing after my time in Indonesia. It did mean, however, I was often away and not able to train or play football regularly, so I started taking my running shoes along when I travelled to run and keep fit. My wife watched with amusement my change. When I did the race that year, she did the four-kilometre walk event, but she watched the runners pass by in the thousands each sweating, puffing but proud of their efforts to complete the race. She must have been thinking she can do better than walk four kilometres.

On New Year's Eve there is a tradition to set resolutions. People typically resolve to get fitter, drink less, lose weight, get a promotion and most, if not all resolutions, fade away within a few weeks. This time Maria stated she would not only run the 12- kilometre City to Surf race in August but that she would run it in under an hour averaging less than five minutes per kilometre. There were a few snickers around the room, but I knew that if she set her mind to it, she would get back into the form that she had twenty years previously in Indonesia. Since the age of thirty, she had completed a diploma in Accounting, a Bachelor degree in Commerce and her Certified Practising Accountant qualifications all while raising four children and working for part of the time, so I knew if she set her mind to it, she would do it.

The next Monday was her first training run and on went the running shoes. We set out for her first serious run in almost twenty years. I suggested a short 5-kilometre run. It lasted about 800 metres. She suggested we cut back along to the beach and home. It was a total of approximately 2 kilometres and some involved walking, but it was a good start. I reminded her that she was still beating everyone who was sitting on their couch. It also reminded me of the Confucius quote from 2 500 years ago.

'The man who moves a mountain begins
by carrying small stones'.

The very next day she could hardly walk down the stairs as her thigh muscles were hurting so much, but so began her renewed running career.

As the days went by and days turned into weeks and the weeks into months the training continued. Two kilometres became three. A run turned into one that you could stop when you liked, so a 4-kilometre run was made up of segments of running and walking then running and less walking then just running for 5 kilometres. I knew then that averaging five minutes per kilometre over 12 kilometres was a challenging task, but she kept going and 5-kilometre runs turned into slow 10-kilometre runs, then faster runs. It was then that she decided it was the shoes that were too slow. So, we went to the running store and looked for better fitting shoes and socks that did not have creases which cause blisters. These are all the things that a new budding runner looks for, especially one that is aiming for a faster time than last.

Around month five of her eight-month training journey, Maria was comfortably completing the 12-kilometre run every week, although at a slow pace, too slow for her liking and her goal. She would also do three other 5-kilometre runs during each week totalling four runs and 27 kilometres each week. At this point she went for a 5-kilometre run with our son Elliot who raced her around the 5-kilometre path. She ran and ran and finished the 5-kilometre loop in 23 minutes. So, she could run at the five-minutes-per-kilometre pace for 5 kilometres, and at least that was a milestone.

Most runners who want to improve often reach for magazines or books to get inspiration. One author came back to mind from my long-forgotten past. It was James Fixx. My father had lent me his book many years ago. James, or Jim as he was known, had written the bestselling book *The Complete Book of Running* in 1977. It's believed his book helped popularise the sport of running and demonstrated the health benefits of regular running not just in the United States but globally. I recall in his second book entitled *Jim Fixx's Second Book of Running* the opening section described a runner doing interval training by running along a path and for one gap between two light poles he would sprint as fast as he could. Then he would run slower between the next two light poles and repeat both paces for the run. Maria and I thought this was an excellent and simple way to do interval training once per week. I subsequently realised many years later, when I bought a heart rate monitor and learned more about the use of the monitor that the aim was to get your heart rate up into the red zone which for us was over 160 beats per minute over that 30 minute period and this would help increase your stamina, speed and fitness.

So, Maria and I started this type of interval training. We did a one-kilometre run to warm up and then did the interval training for four kilometres and a slight warm-down. Well that was the theory. In practice, we did four lots of sprints and were exhausted and ran slowly home on our first run. Later that week we repeated the same exercise with the same result. However, the next week we did six lots of sprints and we continued until we managed to do the sprints each second light pole all the way along the four-kilometre track. We were making progress and Maria's and my times were improving.

Finally, the time came for the race. We lined up early in the cool morning air in August with the large group of nervous runners on St Georges Terrace in Perth. We agreed to not run together but to run our own race. During the race I passed an old friend and colleague of mine called Steve. He was a lovely guy who, while not a regular runner, was still fit and running at a nice pace. He waved and we agreed to contact each other the following week. I arrived at the beachside finish line in 53 minutes or 4.4 minutes per kilometre which was okay for the hilly course. I waited at the finish line with the family for Maria to come in.

Fifty-six minutes passed, then fifty-seven. Fifty-eight minutes ticked by. We were worried that something may have gone wrong. Did she fall over or have some other mishap? The clock ticked over fifty-nine minutes and we then saw her turn into the final straight about 200 metres away with her head down, obviously exhausted, but determined to beat the clock that was located immediately over the white archway of the finish line. Down she came one foot after another, the strain as obvious on her face as the determination in her eyes. You could sense her lungs were burning, her breaths labouring and her legs weakening with each step. She crossed the line with fourteen seconds to go. She did it, met her goal and slumped onto the grass just past the finish line exhausted, trying to hold back the tears of emotion as they trickled out down her cheeks. More importantly, she rediscovered her confidence and her love of running. She had then commenced a fascinating running journey that would last for a long time, take her all over the world and onto finisher podiums in faraway remote places.

Later that week I flew overnight to Tokyo. It was a nine-and-a-half-hour flight to Tokyo. Most times I managed eight hours sleep by the time I arrived early in the morning. I was a good sleeper on planes. I travelled to Japan on business ten times a year back then, so this was a regular trip. After the flight I bought a coffee from Starbucks in the train station below the airport and caught the Narita Express train into the city. As this was in the early 2000s it was not easy to get emails when you were away from the office. Wi-fi and the Blackberry phone were not available then nor were any of the smartphones like the iPhone. The iPhone was not launched until 2007.

So when I got to the hotel early in the morning from the Tokyo train station via the Marunouchi subway line, the first thing I normally did was try to connect back to my office to get the emails that had been coming in over the weekend. To connect I had to disconnect the phone line from the back of the hotel room phone and plug it into my laptop computer. I then had to start up a remote access software, put in a special phone number for Japan connections, and then I would connect the computer back to my office in Australia. I needed a special code plus a secret code that I received by a key fob that I carried with me. Often, I couldn't always get access but when I did it was a frustrating process that could take thirty minutes or more. In 2020 you would just turn on your smartphone. Thank you, Apple Inc and Steve Jobs.

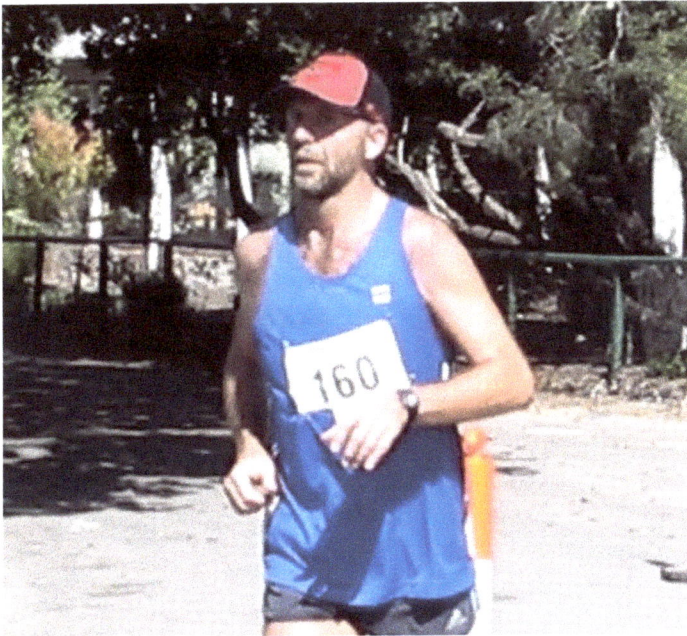

Steve

That morning I was lucky. I got straight into the office network and started downloading my emails. Among the piles of emails was a message from Steve with whom I briefly chatted during the City to Surf race on the weekend. It was short, as is his way. It said, 'Great to see you on the weekend. Do you want to run a marathon in October on Rottnest Island?' I was always up for some fun and a challenge, so I replied 'Hi Steve, sure that's a great idea. Please count me in.' The next thing I did was google 'What is a marathon?' and then 'marathon training program'.

> *'Do not be afraid to go out on a limb*
> *— that is where the fruit is.'*
> Anonymous

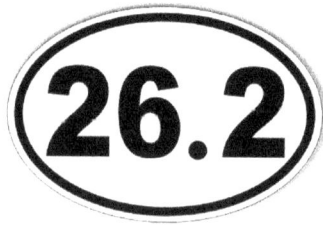

Chapter 4

Running Rotto

The name marathon comes from the herb fennel and there's a town in Greece which is so named as there was an abundance of fennel plants in the area. It's a small town of around 13 000 people now and it's located on a small plain near the east coast. In ancient times the Athenians had a famous battle there with the Persians in 490 BC called the Battle of Marathon. After the Greek forces defeated the Persians, who were led by Darius, the Persians set sail for Athens to attack the unprotected city. The Athenians marched the army back to Athens to do just that. There are numerous legends linked with the battle and one legend is that a Greek messenger, Pheidippides ran approximately 26 miles from the battlefield at Marathon to Athens in order to relay news of the victory and warn the city that the Persians were on their way by ship. According to legend he only said, 'We were victorious!' collapsed, and died from exhaustion.

There is, however, a debate on the accuracy of this story. The Greek historian Herodotus mentions a Philippides, not Pheidippides, who ran as a messenger from Athens to Sparta to ask for help, and then he ran back covering 250 kilometres (150 miles) each way. The original games which took place in Greece around 776 BC to 393 AD did not have a marathon race. However, when the first modern Olympics were being planned the organisers looked for a significant event which would have roots in the ancient history of Greece and selected this run by Pheidippides from the town of Marathon to Athens. The first Olympic marathon was won by Spyridon Louis in two hours fifty-eight minutes and fifty seconds in 1896 and was run over 40 kilometres (approximately 25 miles). The Boston Marathon began a year later, on the 19th April 1897, as the Boston Athletics Association was inspired by the success of the first marathon competition in the 1896 Summer Olympics. The Boston marathon is run in April each year and is the oldest annually run marathon event. Females could participate for the first time in 1972.

The marathon has been in each summer Olympics since 1896. In the 1908 games, the length of the race was extended. The games were being held in London and according to some, Princess Mary requested that the race commence on the lawn of Windsor Castle, which is the royal residence in the English county of Berkshire. The race finish was in front of the King in the royal box at the

White City Olympic Stadium in London. This distance was 42.195 kilometres (26.2 miles), and the distance became standardised in 1921. So, the modern marathon is 42.195 kilometres or 26.2 miles because a princess wanted it to start in one place and the organisers wanted it to finish at the stadium in front of the royal box.

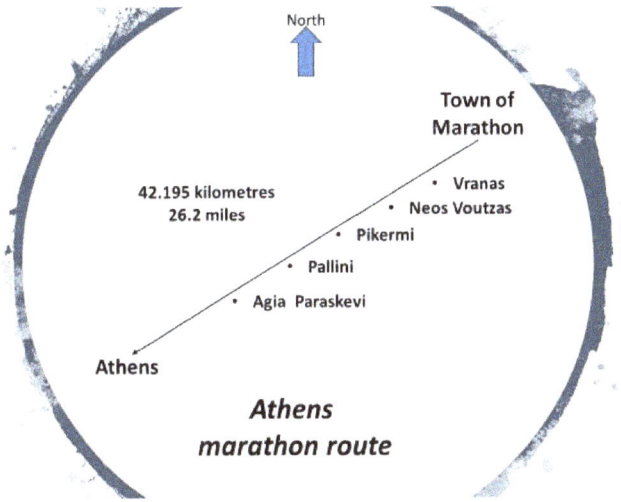

Athens marathon route

That's a long way. The longest distance I had run up to this point was twelve kilometres and even twelve kilometres was a very long run for me. I had never thought of running that far at one time let alone in a race. It was daunting and I did feel nervous, but I made a commitment to Steve so I would follow through. I was also excited to have this new goal, and even though I had never run that distance before, I never thought that I would not start nor would I fail to finish.

'Successful people build each other up.
They motivate, inspire, and push each other.'
— Anonymous

The next Google search I did after the message from Steve was to search for a basic marathon training program and key marathon training tips as I only had ten weeks to prepare. That made me nervous.

The key tips I took away from my reading were:

- No excuses.
- Always get a medical check-up before embarking on an exercise program.
- If you get injured, stop running and rest until you have recovered.
- To reduce the risk of injury, build your total running distance each week slowly.
- The aim is to not increase your weekly total run distance by more than ten per cent each week. I thought that a ten per cent increase each week was doable.
- Do a long run once a week and do shorter runs on days during the week.
- Ideally, build your long run up to a 30 kilometre distance and repeat this length at least three times at the back end of your training immediately prior to the final week of training for a marathon.
- Taper in the last week of your training prior to the race.

- Have at least one rest day a week.
- Try and do interval training once per week to get your heart rate up into the red zone. Typically, this meant high intensity runs of 200, 400, 800 or 1200 metres with a rest in between each run over a total of five kilometres in each weekly session. This normally takes only thirty minutes.
- Hydrate well and during the longer runs consume some high energy foods e.g. Medjool dates, every thirty minutes.
- Buy good, well-fitting shoes which are half a size too big to reduce the risk of losing toenails and buy socks which are reasonably tight fitting as creases in your socks cause blisters; and
- Every four or five weeks reduce your total distance to help recovery.

I liked the 'no excuses' point the most. I found once I set my mind to something I would follow through. That is why I always write down my goals. They become a commitment. When my dad decided that he would go running every morning at 5.30 I went with him. There were no excuses like it was too early, too cold or I was too tired. When it came to study there were always times in each semester when a suitable excuse would pop up. Maybe it was an illness or a work commitment, but I always came back to the 'no excuses' rule. So, my fit with this statement in running was a good one. It was about not letting obstacles get in my way, always being positive and optimistic, and not looking for a reason to avoid a commitment.

The medical check-up is critical. People do die during strenuous exercise, and later in my running races and triathlons, athletes died in the races I entered. So, it's always important to get that medical check-up before starting an exercise program. I always have an annual medical check-up with my physician. Don't become so focused on the start and finish lines to the point you ignore your personal safety.

The training schedule I chose was to use 40 kilometres each week as my base as I had been doing that prior to the City to Surf race.

- Week one — four by 10-kilometre runs per week as the base.
- Week two — increase by ten per cent to 44 kilometres
- Four by 10-kilometre runs during the week plus a short 4-kilometre run on Sunday.
- I used Sunday as the one day I would increase my distance. It could also have been any other day like a Saturday.
- I set two rest days — Friday and Monday.
- Week three — increase by ten per cent to 48 kilometres.
- Four 10-kilometre runs, and an 8-kilometre run on Sunday.

- Week four — four 10-kilometre runs, and a 13-kilometre run on Sunday.
- Week five — four 10-kilometre runs, and an 18-kilometre run on Sunday.
- Week six — four 10-kilometre runs, and a 24-kilometre run on Sunday.
- Week seven — four 10-kilometre runs, and the first 30-kilometre run.
- Week eight — four 10-kilometre runs, and 30-kilometre run on Sunday.
- Week nine — four 10-kilometre runs, and 30-kilometre run on Sunday.
- Week ten — two 10-kilometre runs and a short final run of 4 kilometres two days before the race. On the day before the race I would do a 3-kilometre walk.

After all this I realised the truth in the quote:

'All roads that lead to success have to pass through hard work boulevard at some point.'
— Anonymous

The program I selected was basic. It was designed to get enough distance into my training and build up as per my plan at no more than ten per cent per week. If someone had a lower initial base of weekly runs the build-up would take longer. My plan also met my goal to do the marathon in ten weeks. I didn't do any interval training and I did all the runs at a nice comfortable pace, not slow, but not stretching my limits. Sometimes if I was exhausted, I would walk and when I felt better, I would start to run again. I felt that there was nothing wrong with walking. I called it the 'walk of common sense' not the 'walk of shame'. It was better to stop, walk a bit and restart when I felt like it than to keep pushing myself. I knew that my fitness would keep improving and in time I could run all the distance without walking. It was better to get to the starting line than train beyond my limits and injure myself. I had measured out a five-kilometre route from my home and I could simply repeat it for ten kilometres. I also measured out a ten-kilometre distance in Bold Park which is near to my home as an alternative route. I like to keep running simple, so I run without any music as I like to enjoy the scenery wherever I run even if it is in the centre of a big city.

Sunday was my long run day. I don't know why I did that but for me it was the day when I had the most available time. I worked all week so I could fit in an hour run in the evenings and Saturdays were normally busy doing household jobs like gardening so that left Sunday. On the long runs, typically, I would ask my wife, Maria, to drive me at a suitable time the set distance from the house. I remember for my first 30- kilometre run we were away from home staying in the north of Busselton for the weekend and Maria drove me 30 kilometres down the coast from where we were staying to Dunsborough. For me it was a long, long drive which seemed to never end. I nervously stepped out of the car wondering if I would ever be able to run the 30 kilometres back. The family waited back at the house where we were staying and wondered if I would ever return, but sure enough three and a half hours later, I arrived back. I was tired, dusty, and thirsty but happy that my training was on track. I was also happy that I was able to run that far without any injury or exhaustion. It also made me less nervous about completing the marathon.

Many times when people asked Maria or me about running and training, a comment would often follow along the lines of 'I don't have time to train' or ' I am just too busy to exercise'. I even had a comment once from a work colleague which was 'don't you have a few (alcoholic) drinks when you get home from work every day?' When I hear this, I think of the well-known but anonymous quote:

'If you want to get something done, give it to a busy person.'

This quote, although anonymous, has been ascribed to many people like Lucille Ball, Benjamin Franklin, Elbert Hubbard, or even WJ Kennedy but I like the quote because it's true. Busy people manage their time. They schedule in the important things and just get things done. What do we do? We watch very little television. That frees up the evenings as we don't have any 'favourite TV programs'.

- We read the news, weather, stock market news and other things briefly on the internet.
- Prior to the internet we read the newspaper briefly in the morning.
- I decided to simply get up thirty minutes earlier each day, so it gave me extra time to be well organised and ready for the day.
- We discuss, agree, and write down our annual goals so we both know that what we agreed on is important. This avoids distractions and time wasters.
- When we had four children we also worked and studied so scheduling in important things was vital as well as scheduling out the unimportant.

When our children were still at school, we took the time to take them to all sorts of training and sports events, take active roles as coaches, umpires, referees as well as committee members to help keep the clubs running.

During that ten weeks I still travelled three times to Asia. On one trip to Tokyo I went out to dinner with four Japanese customers. Takafumi, who was a Tokyo-based colleague, was with me and we all discussed my planned marathon. They were impressed as the Japanese I worked with were always respectful and appreciative. They decided that we should take bets on how long I would take to finish the race. The bets ranged from four to five hours.

My colleague collected the bets and they left excited to see what time I would finish in.

When I travelled it was still important to keep up the training schedule. 'No excuses.' I found it especially challenging as I didn't like doing morning runs. I preferred to run in the evening when my body was warmed up. I normally stayed at a hotel close to the centre of Tokyo near to the Tokyo railway station and the Imperial Palace. The Imperial Palace includes the residence of the emperor, together with three palace sanctuaries and the headquarters of the Imperial Household. It was built on the site of the Edo Castle complex during the Edo period (1603-1868). Fortunately for me, the distance around the Imperial Palace is approximately five kilometres and it's a very popular, safe, and beautiful place for people in Tokyo to run. I used this every evening to do my training runs. In fact, I felt privileged to be able to run around the palace in the evenings. If I had a customer dinner I would run after dinner so sometimes I could be found running at 11 pm or midnight and there would always be other people running no matter what time of the night. I remember running there several times in spring when the cherry blossoms were out and running under the cherry trees up near the British Embassy. Even the Japanese Crown Prince Naruhito has been seen running in the vicinity.

Similarly, if I was to visit Taipei, I would run down to the Chiang Kai-shek Memorial Hall which is a famous national monument and landmark in the Zhongzheng district. It was erected in memory of Generalissimo Chiang Kai-shek who was the former President of the Republic of China. The white building is impressive, with four sides and a blue octagonal roof. There are two sets of stairs and each has eighty-nine steps which represents Chiang Kai-shek's age when he died. When I went there, I would run up the main steps on the outside the building in place of my dismissed interval training. I would repeat this ten times and then continue my run. Over the years I mapped out running routes in all the main cities I visited on business especially Tokyo, Seoul, Shanghai, Singapore, London, and Denver.

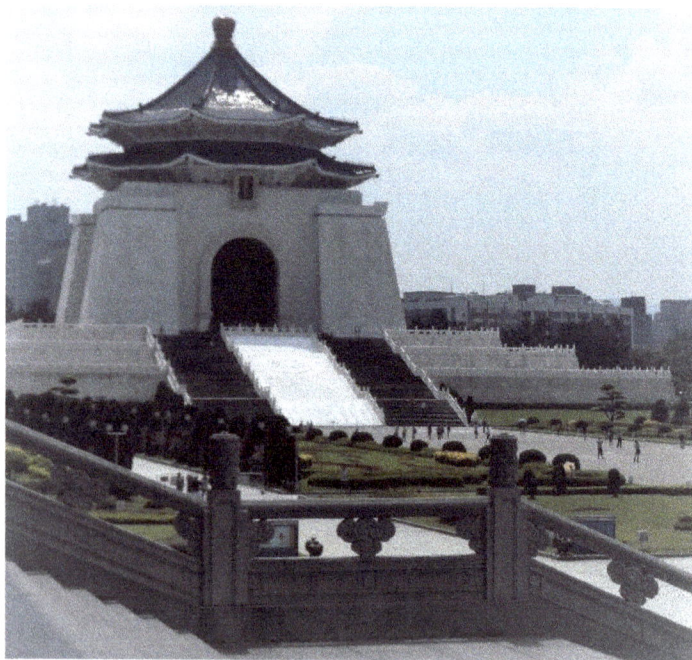

Chiang Kai-shek Memorial Hall — Taipei, Taiwan

In Shanghai, the running route depended on where I was staying. I have stayed at the fabulous Peace Hotel on the Bund which is a promenade along the Huangpu River. A run around that historical area in the evening or early morning is fascinating with the display of traditional housing combined with the ultra-modern towering buildings across the river in Pudong.

In London it's easy to run as there are so many amazing places in the downtown area. For me it was like I was given the wonderful opportunity to do a tour of London each morning. Normally I would stay in one of two areas. One was in Paddington, adjacent to the historic Paddington railway station where our office was located, and the other was near St James's Square on Regent Street. The routes of choice were to either run from Paddington out past Little Venice along the canal past the numerous low canal boats and back or down across Bayswater Road to the Lancaster Gate entrance of Hyde Park and down the path inside the park to Kensington Gardens. At Kensington Gardens I would normally run down past the palace and Round Pond and just before Kensington Grove turn left onto the path past The Albert Memorial. At the end of the path at Hyde Park Corner I would either turn left up Park Lane past Marble Arch back to the hotel or if I wanted a longer run I would cross to Wellington Arch and go down Constitution Hill past Buckingham Palace up The Mall through Admiralty Arch and then track through Trafalgar Square and Piccadilly Circus across Mayfair back to Paddington. Some mornings I would do an even longer run and cross St James's Park to Westminster, across the Westminster Bridge and down along the Thames River to London Bridge across the bridge and back to Paddington.

I would often pause and look at the statue of Captain Cook on the right-hand side of The Mall as he was the first English ship captain to land on and map the east coast of Australia. Buckingham Palace also captured my attention as I ran around the roundabout. I would always take a small detour and stop on St James's Square at a small memorial for Yvonne Fletcher. She was a Metropolitan Police officer who was fatally wounded at that location in April 1984 by a shot fired from the Libyan Embassy on St James's Square. The gunman remains unknown. She was simply deployed to monitor a demonstration outside the Libyan embassy. That memorial, for some reason captivated me as she seemed to be a lovely woman senselessly shot in the prime of life. Every time I would stop and pay my respects to her. Oddly enough, I now have a grandson named Fletcher.

I must confess that sometimes I could get obsessive with my running training program so much so that if I scheduled a run, I felt I must run. No excuses. One morning in London I stayed at a hotel on Piccadilly across from Green Park in the middle of winter. I rose earlier than six in the morning because of jet lag as I would work with the jet lag rather than against it. Some mornings

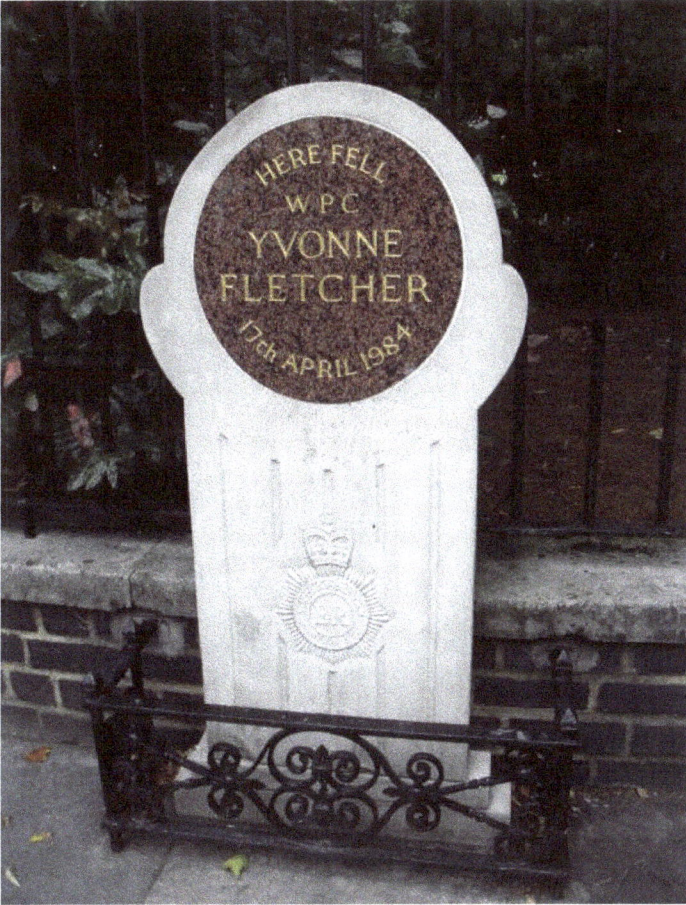

that week it was dark and cold with frost on the ground in Hyde Park, but I still ran. I loved running around Hyde Park and Kensington Gardens early in the morning as they are such beautiful, historic, peaceful, easy places to run. One morning however, when I got to the foyer of the hotel, I could see it was snowing so I walked out onto the edge of the road and stood in the snow with snow falling all around me. I stood there for a full five minutes looking up and down the road wondering if it was safe to run. After much contemplation I sadly turned around and went back into the hotel after deciding that it would be unsafe to run. The snow would cover up any dangerous potholes in the trails and the ice would be slippery. As I walked back into the foyer, I saw a colleague of mine sitting in a high-backed lounge chair smoking a cigarette, staring at me. The smoke swirled about him. He must have been observing me for quite some time while I stood outside in my shorts and sweatshirt in the snow. His morning greeting summed up his conclusions about my mental state, 'You're fucking mad!'

After the ten weeks of training it came time for the big test, the marathon on Rottnest Island. Little did I know at the time that this would be marathon number one of thirty! Rottnest or Rotto as the locals call the island is a beautiful small island 18 kilometres (11 miles) off the coast of Perth in Western Australia.

It's a sandy, low lying island formed with a base of limestone and surrounded by beautiful sandy beaches and a crystal-clear blue-green sea. It's a protected A-class reserve and is home to the Quokka, which is a famous small, wallaby like marsupial on the island that appears to be unafraid of people. According to history, the Dutch mariner Samuel Volckertzoon documented the sighting of 'a wild rat' on Rottnest Island in 1658. In 1696, Willem de Vlamingh mistook the Quokkas for giant rats and named the island 'Rotte nest', which still stands today.

There are thousands of these native marsupials around the island. The Quokka now features prominently on every finisher's medal with the Latin words *Veni Vidi Vici*.

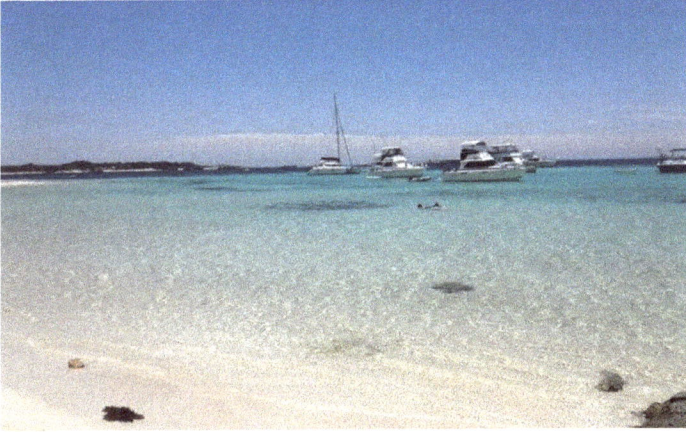

Rottnest Island

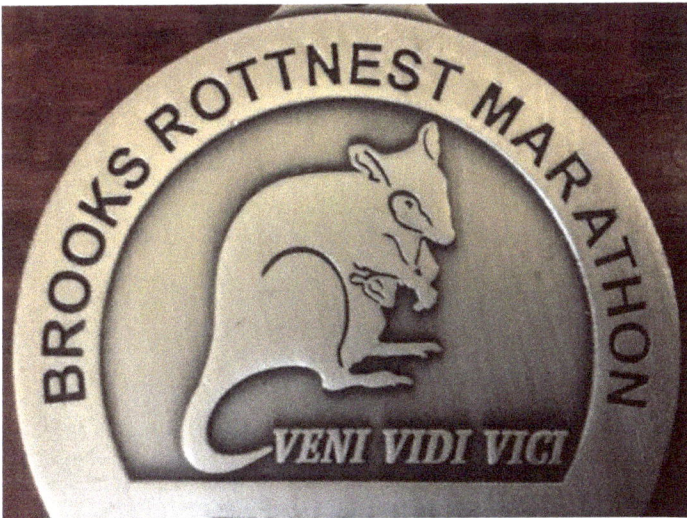

Rottnest Island Medal
'I came, I saw, I conquered.' — Julius Caesar — 47 BC

The island covers 19 square kilometres (7.3 square miles). It has a small permanent population of 300 people with around 500 000 annual visitors and regular ferry schedule to and from the coastal cities of Perth and Fremantle. A permanent settlement was established there in 1829 and has hosted a penal colony, military installation, internment camps for enemy aliens and more recently in 2020 a place to isolate some travellers coming into Australia from overseas. This was one of the Covid-19 virus epidemic isolation processes used in Western Australia to isolate people for fourteen days. Many of the current buildings date back to the colonial period and are now tourist accommodation. The island also has modern facilities like a resort, golf course, tennis courts, hotel, restaurants, and a village.

Each year now it has a running festival on a Sunday including 5-kilometre, 10- kilometre, half-marathon and full marathon races. The first marathon was run in 1994. As the island is relatively small the marathon consists of four loops starting in the village and circumnavigating the salt lakes in the centre of the island running out along the available roads up to a small hill and past someone playing the bagpipes. The races were held each year in October after the winter rains are finished and before the heat of summer sets in.

We arrived the night before and stayed in apartment accommodation on the island. It was a short walk to the start of the race. My family had come over to be my cheer squad and my wife promised to run the last few kilometres with me. Steve was there and said he had done his training. Some of his family were there as well. This was a new experience for everyone as the distance was daunting and the temperature expected to be 30 degrees Celsius (86 °F) so it was like going into the unknown, but we had done the training so we felt slightly confident. I had completed three 30-kilometre runs and kept to my running schedule. Steve was expecting a time around four and a half hours. I had not set a target, but I thought six minutes per kilometre or four hours twelve minutes was possible considering I could run a 10-kilometre (6 mile) race in under five minutes per kilometre. We decided to run our own race and catch up at the finish.

During the evening prior to the race the organisers arranged what was called a 'Carbo Loading' evening for the runners. This essentially was a pasta meal where a variety of pastas were provided to the runners because pasta is high in carbohydrates. One of the organisers explained to me that carbohydrate loading is the process of maximising your muscle glycogen stores by consuming a large quantity of carbohydrate before endurance exercise. At this stage of my marathon experience we decided not to attend the 'Carbo Loading' meal, but we appreciated that the organisers went to the trouble to stage the event. We ate a normal meal in the apartment and had an early night. Over the years we simply did the same. In the morning I had a banana before the race and a cup of coffee.

As I stood at the starting line the following morning, I stretched my legs to get myself ready and to provide me with something to do while waiting. I was nervous. I had butterflies in my stomach as I had never run this far before, but in the pale light of pre- dawn, I never thought I wouldn't finish. I wasn't prone to injury, so I didn't expect to strain a hamstring muscle, slip into a pothole, or collide with another runner. Cramps were a possibility as it was hot, so I reminded myself to take in water and electrolytes at the water stations. However, I knew I could finish.

The run started at what is called 'the village' which is a small settlement on the island that provided food, groceries and other services for visitors and locals. The road was shaded by beautiful tall trees and adjacent to a small park called Heritage Common where the race would finish and the celebrations would be held. I looked over to the park and saw the colourful banners and archway identifying the marathon finishing line. I thought in four hours plus I would be there. I wished Steve all the best with a handshake. I don't know why we did that, but it seemed like an offer of respect to each other for doing all the training and daring to show up to do the race.

Just before the race started bagpipes began to play the wonderful tune 'Amazing Grace' to set the scene for the day ahead. The race has its own mythology. The legend has it that Harry McFordyce, who was an immigrant prisoner on Rottnest Island many years ago, escaped the hands of justice and attempted to run off the island. On the fourth circuit around the island McFordyce succumbed to dehydration and died, or so the myth goes. When you run the marathon, participants see and hear the ghost of Harry playing his bagpipes on top of the hill overlooking Armstrong Bay.

The first two laps of the four-lap circuit went easily as it was a relatively flat course, shaded in parts and open to bright sunlight in others. Part of the race went around the salt lakes of Government House Lake, the longer Serpentine Lake, Lake Vincent, and Herschel Lake. These used to be used for commercial salt production in the long distant past but now are sanctuaries for thousands of birds and other wildlife. Even though the race started early in the morning, by this time at nine o'clock the temperature was reaching the expected 30 degrees. The number of people running the race was small so by the end of the second lap all the runners were spread out over the course. I briefly chatted with one runner who was doing the run as a bet he made with a friend just the week before the race. He was a former Ironman triathlete and was convinced he could do the marathon without any training. He finished in under four hours. Another runner was a recovered heart transplant patient who carefully trained for the event with his physicians' guidance and wanted to just show people that even if life puts significant challenges in one's path, we can overcome them. No excuses. He finished in good time as well.

I slowed my pace in the third lap but was pleased to see the man playing the bagpipes on top of the hill. That meant the remainder of that lap was mostly downhill. The race organisers had a few novelties which played out during the race. On the last lap at the foot of Harry's Hill I was given a gold coin by the 'dollar girls'. They were young ladies who dressed up as Cat Woman, Super Woman, Wonder Woman, or in another fancy dress, and they gave us a gold dollar coin to pay the piper who stood a few hundred metres up at the top of the hill playing the bagpipes. So, on the last circuit, we would throw the dollar coin into the piper's hat, hence the term 'pay the piper'. Legend says failure to pay the piper would result in cramps, dehydration or another tragedy imposed on you by the ghost of Harry. I'm not superstitious but I felt I needed all the help I could get so I paid the piper not to incur Harry's wrath.

The family waited at a set point at the halfway point on each lap. It was so good to get the cheers and encouragement. As I was new to marathon running, I took along some tubes of corn starch which I bought from the running store in town. They seemed to work. I ate part of one every thirty minutes which boosted my energy and enthusiasm. The lesson I learned, however, was that when you sweat in the heat of the day, food can turn into a sticky mess in your pocket.

Finally, I went into the fourth and final lap. I felt drained at this point. Sweat was pouring down my face and my shirt was soaked. As it was hot the sweat dried on my legs leaving a faint dusting of salt making my legs look white. When I passed the family, Maria started the run with me on the last half of the final lap. I recall trudging up one of the long slow hills and she was springing along having fun laughing and sometimes running backwards for fun. As I turned into the final straight past the old colonial villages and the village, I looked at the clock above the finish line and it read four hours and four minutes or just under the six minute per kilometre mark. I was absolutely exhausted after such an extreme event. It was such a relief to finish. Steve came in a little later at four hours and eighteen minutes. We were presented with our marathon finisher medal, grabbed a cold drink and a banana, and then headed down to the beach to soak our run weary legs and wash away the sweat in the cool refreshing ocean water and reminisce about our first marathon.

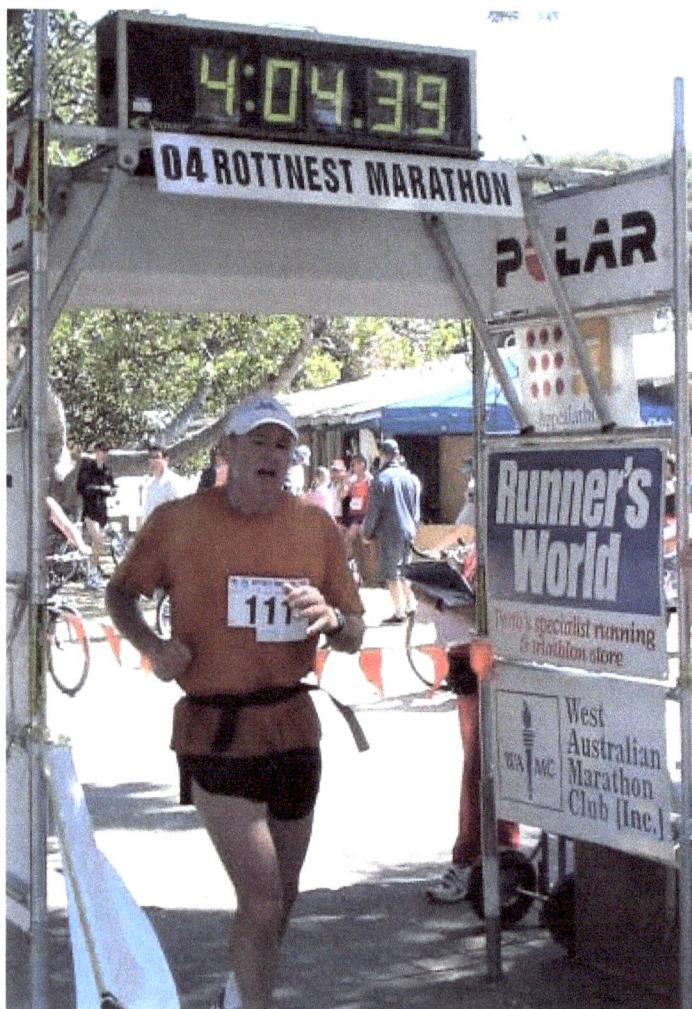

Rottnest marathon — 2004

'A marathon is like life with its ups and downs, but once you have done it, you feel that you can do anything if you put your mind to it.'
— Anonymous

Chapter 5

On holidays,
I plan to run a marathon

My first marathon was over just like that. During the following week, my mind came around to the following conclusions. The first was that both training and the race were demanding, challenging, and exhausting. I wasn't convinced that I should do a second one. It was a significant commitment. The second thought was that because I had done the training according to my plan, I didn't have any injuries or pain following the run. Immediately after the run I was stiff in the muscles, but I recovered quickly. So, proper training, conditioning, nutrition, and hydration seemed to be the key. I think having a lean physique was also important. The third point came from my friend Peter who said he loved doing the training for an endurance event because once you finish all the preparation you feel physically in top shape and fantastic. It did feel incredible to be really fit, lean and confident.

The other point I thought about was that during a typical run it would start off slow, a bit painful with laboured breaths, but as I got into the training I would run freer, faster and get a bit of what is called a runner's high in a run. This is often described as a feeling of euphoria that's believed to be associated with the release of endorphins by the brain. These endorphins are reported to be released during long, continuous workouts of moderate to high intensity with physical stress. Strangely enough for me I enjoyed the running and the good feeling that went with in. That didn't mean I didn't feel exhausted in my early days of training, but after I got fitter, I often didn't feel the pain. I would go on a long run and enjoy it. After thirty minutes of high-intensity interval training, I would very often feel euphoric.

The next year Maria and I continued as normal except Maria decided that she too wanted to do a marathon. There were no muffled laughs this time as the family all knew if she set her mind to it, she would do it. I would be her training partner, so I reasoned I was locked into doing a second marathon!

We developed a training program together. The training was simply for us and not intended as a guide for anyone else. Over the years we've read several articles and books related to running. Many people have also been very generous in providing their advice, lending books to us or buying books for us. I even received a book for Christmas titled *Running & Philosophy — A Marathon for the Mind*, edited by Michael W Austin. Who knew people wrote on this topic? I enjoyed the book, particularly the chapter 'Chasing Happiness Together: Running and Aristotle's Philosophy of Friendship'. I also read a book by Dean Karnazes titled *50 Marathons 50 Days — The Secret to Super Endurance*. The message there for me was that even great endurance athletes struggle and must do the work and be determined to succeed.

Even after all the reading and experimenting we don't propose that we are experts in the field, just that we have developed a training plan that worked for us to become competent runners. For elite runners, their programs are very different, and they get a different set of results. Many professional athletes do their training on a full-time basis or study / work part-time and train full-time. Their training is much more scientific and includes at least two training sessions a day. People must get proper medical advice and a medical check-up before engaging in any physical activity like this and then read widely, take advice, listen carefully, and develop a program that suits them. For those who feel more comfortable with a coach there are many running coaches, and many are professional physical therapists as well as runners. They have a wide range of processes including scientific computer programs to guide every level of runner from beginner to professional.

Here is the simple training plan we use.

Basic training plan

Stage one — building the base fitness for running

1. If you have not run before, remember the ten per cent rule and start off with walking and some running, then build your program into a run / walk each day for five days per week. Increase your weekly distance by only ten per cent per week.

2. Build to run 5 km for five days per week at a nice steady pace. Remember you can walk whenever you feel you need to.

3. Try for two rest days each week. One on Friday before a club race* on Saturday and one on Monday so you have a rest day after the Sunday longer run.

4. For longer runs take water and something to eat e.g. two or three Medjool dates and eat one every thirty minutes.

5. A weekly run with a running club is good as it's a time to run with other people.

6. Running in the morning, lunchtime or evening is optional. Whatever works for you.

7. Start increasing the Sunday distance by 2 km each week up to 15 km: and

8. Try a half-marathon race at a nice steady pace once you get to a regular 15 km on a Sunday.

*A weekly club run is a good idea as it puts you in a

competitive race each week. Parkrun is a good run to do. It was founded by Paul Sinton-Hewitt in 2004 at Bushy Park in London, England. It is now a worldwide network of free, timed 5-kilometre runs which are typically held on a Saturday morning.

Stage two – building up the pace and fitness

1. Continue running 5 km for five days per week with the 15 km longer run on a Sunday.
2. Interval training — add in one day per week a set of interval training during a normal 5 km run.

   ✦ After a 1-km warm-up sprint between two light poles, then jog for the next two light poles, then sprint between the next two light poles. Warm up 1 km, 3 km interval training, 1 km cool-down.

   ✦ Another alternative is to find a nice hill of 400 metres length and after a warm-up (five minutes), run at pace up the hill and jog or walk down — repeat for twenty minutes and five-minute cool-down.

   ✦ Another alternative is to find a football field and after a warm-up (five minutes), run at pace around 400 metres and jog the next 400 metres — repeat for twenty minutes and five-minute cool-down.

   ✦ At any time, it is OK to walk as you build up your fitness.

- ✦ The aim is to do no more than thirty minutes of interval training each week so after a time the aim is to do a 500 metre warm-up and cool-down with 4 km of intervals.

3. Consider using a heart rate monitor to try and maintain a heart rate at or above 140 beats per minute during each of the runs after the warm-up. The aim is to increase fitness and endurance.

4. Once this is completed the aim is to do another half-marathon. This is the base level.

5. When the marathon is ten weeks in the future, the aim was to move to the next stage.

Stage three – marathon training stage

1. Week one — Ramp up the daily run distance to 6 km per running day and add an extra 2 km on Sunday (17 km) — 41 km.

2. Week two — Ramp up your daily run distance to 7 km per running day and add on an extra 2 km on Sunday (19 km) — 47 km.

3. Week three — Ramp up your daily run distance to 8 km per running day and add on an extra 2 km on Sunday (21 km) — 53 km.

4. Week four — same as week three — 53 km.

5. Week five — Ramp up your daily run distance to 9 kilometres per running day and add on an extra 2 kilometres on Sunday (23 km) — 59 km.

6. Week six — Ramp up your daily run distance to 10

km per running day and add on an extra 2 km on Sunday (25 km) — 65 km.

7. Week seven — Maintain your daily run distance at 10 km per running day and add a 30 km slow steady run on Sunday — 70 km.

8. Weeks eight and nine — maintain week seven program for two more weeks.

9. Week ten — week before the marathon — do 4–5 km runs with a rest day immediately before the marathon day.

10. Marathon day — get a support team to cheer. Take enough Medjool dates to have one each thirty minutes (60 calories plus enough minerals).

11. In a race water will be supplied so there is no need to carry water. Wear well-fitting socks. Have shoes that are worn in and a half size bigger than normal i.e. room in the toe. Try not to wear a new running shirt (nipple bleeding for men), bring a running cap and wear sunscreen.

12. Remember the aim is not to run fast but at a nice steady pace that is comfortable. The aim is to run your own race. It does not matter about the time.

13. Consider walking through the drink stations for 20 seconds. The aim for this is to conserve your energy and allow you to run better at the latter stages of the race.

14. Enjoy the event.

'Don't try to overhaul your life overnight. Instead, focus on making one small change at a time. Over time, those small changes will add up to a big transformation.'
Anonymous

The reason why I selected Medjool dates was that a friend recommended them to me. They're high in calories and carbohydrates and have some protein but no fat. The sugar in them is usually glucose, fructose and traces of sucrose and maltose plus they are a good source of potassium and copper. They contain around 60 calories each.

Years later I also received some sage advice regarding race preparation. I was competing in the state triathlon championship and after the race the announcer did an 'on air' interview with one of the national triathlon representatives. He asked what her key piece of advice was in preparing for a triathlon competition. She replied that in her view it was personal hygiene. That surprised me and many other people and it grabbed their attention to what she was going to say next. She elaborated that it was obviously critical to do all the training, be motivated, have a good coach and equipment but all of that could be quickly wasted if you got sick. She recommended to:

- wash your hands regularly and thoroughly
- avoid touching things which could be contaminated
- ensure your meals and drinks are from a reliable source

- distance yourself from people (now called social distancing)
- avoid people completely who have cold/flu symptoms
- some other people recommend wearing a face mask when in public.

In Japan, it has been extremely common for people to wear a mask in public long before it became normal with the Covid-19 virus in 2020. In Japan, people who have cold symptoms normally wear a mask to prevent it spreading and other people wear a mask in public to simply not expose themselves to germs from other people. In 2020 this became normal around the world.

We set out a race schedule that year which included two half-marathons in preparation for the Perth marathon and my second attempt at the Rottnest marathon later in the year. Intermingled with this were some 10-kilometre races with the West Australian Marathon Club which held organised races of various lengths on most Sundays at different places within the city. As Maria was doing her first marathon that year she decided to dedicate the run to raise money for the Leukaemia Foundation which provides reliable information on all types of blood cancer as well as the blood cancer journey from diagnosis, to treatment, and beyond for people living with blood cancer, their family members, friends, and health professionals. She felt she was running for a good cause and did raise a significant amount for the charity who were extremely appreciative.

The first test for the year was the Fremantle running festival and the half-marathon (21 kilometres / 13 miles) which I finished in one hour 39 minutes. Steve got excited at my time and it took me a while to realise why. It was 99 minutes, so less than that magical figure of 100 minutes. In the world of a 47-year-old part-time runner, it was a nice, if unexpected, milestone. It was also an average of four minutes and 40 seconds per kilometre. Both Maria and Steve also finished in good times. The Perth half-marathon was next and went well after an anxious start.

Maria and I then had our sights set on the Perth marathon. Steve decided not to participate as he felt at the time one marathon was enough for him. I'm not sure if he ever ran another. The race we did together could have been his first and last marathon. People start running for different reasons and not everyone gets hooked into running and exercise. To stop running and do other exercise is okay too!

One evening in the week before the marathon, I was doing some painting at a property we own and slipped off a small step while painting a wall. I fell awkwardly on my ankle. While I was writhing in the pain of the fall with tears in my eyes, it came to me, I needed to race on the weekend after all that training. So, I packed up my paint equipment as best I could and hobbled home for some RICE treatment.

That is, Rest, Ice, Compression and Elevation treatment. I couldn't walk that evening and rested my ankle for the remainder of the week wondering if I could recover to some state which would allow me to run the 42 kilometres. I recalled my third rule that if I was injured, I would stop training until I recovered. So, I gave myself four days to recover before the run on the weekend.

When Sunday morning arrived, I found I could walk and run with some pain, but it was bearable, so I ignored my third rule, strapped up my ankle and headed off to the starting line with Maria. I had done so much training that I couldn't miss the run. I also remembered my first rule, 'no excuses'. Maria was nervous but ready to run her first marathon. And run she did. The family waited at the finish line and at three hours fifty-three minutes Maria came in running looking just like she had done a short run in the park. The family kept wondering, 'Where is Dad?' as they all expected me to finish before her. A few minutes later I came struggling over the finish line which was adjacent to the beautiful Swan River in Perth near the magnificent Crown Casino. My time was slower at four hours and five minutes, but I finished and didn't give up despite the pain. I found a place in the shade to lie down and let the exhaustion fade away. It took some time! In October that year Maria and I did the Rottnest Marathon with times of 3.54 and 4.09 respectively.

Maria now enjoyed the running and training plus it gave her a unique sense of achievement to complete such a demanding run. So that was marathon number three for me and number two for Maria.

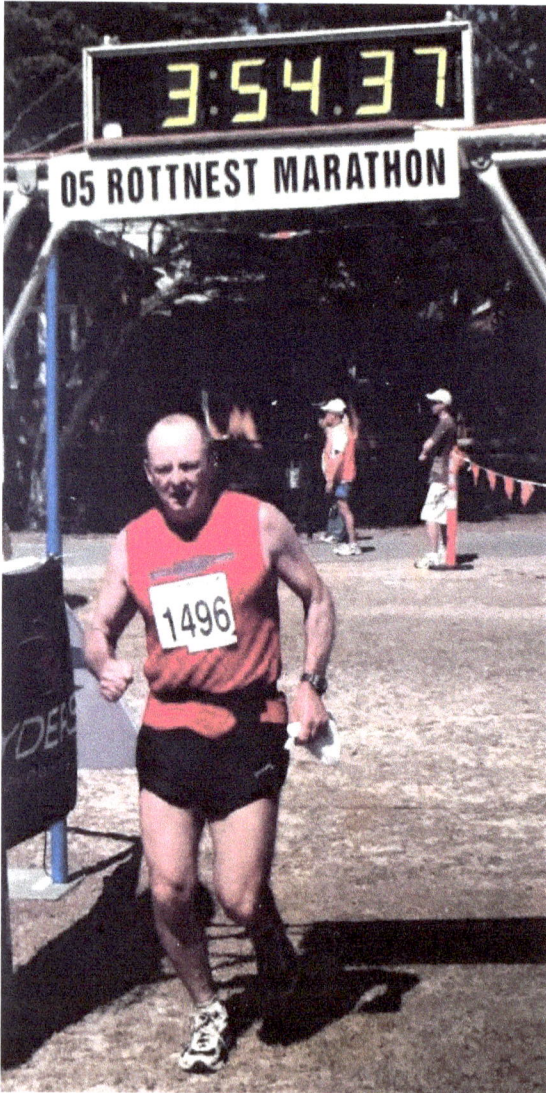

Our final run with Steve for the year was a nice ten-kilometre run around City Beach in Perth. It's often rated as one of Western Australia's best beaches which is not surprising given the golden, clean sandy beach, rolling surf, crystal clear water and beautiful blue sky most of the year. It has always been a pleasure for us to live across the road from the beach and be able to run along the paths there and the adjacent nature wonderlands of Bold Park and Perry Lakes with the many trails, fauna, and flora. As we were running along, Steve told us that he and his family were going to move to Mongolia for work which was a big surprise to us. We also had our own surprise as Maria and I were moving to Singapore to live. We didn't know it at the time, but it was to become our home for the next five and a half years and one of the few times we would see Steve again. His simple message led to a series of amazing adventures for many years to come.

'Sail away from the safe harbour.
Catch the trade winds in your sails.
Explore. Dream. Discover.'
Mark Twain

Singapura — land of the Merlion

The Republic of Singapore is a sovereign city-state and island country located in Southeast Asia just to the south of Malaysia and adjacent to Indonesia. It lies about 137 kilometres (85 miles) north of the equator. The country's territory has one main island with 63 satellite islands. The main island is approximately 40 kilometres (25 miles) by 20 kilometres (12.5 miles) in size and is home to 5.6 million residents. It's densely populated but like Tokyo it's well organised, has excellent public transport and is friendly and safe. The country has four official languages: English, Malay, Chinese, and Tamil with English being the common language between most Singaporeans.

The Merlion is one of the symbols of Singapore. The lion head depicts a lion (singa) and city (pura) while the fish tail symbolises the fishing village of 'Temasek'. The legend is that the Merlion would visit to guard Lion City's wellbeing.

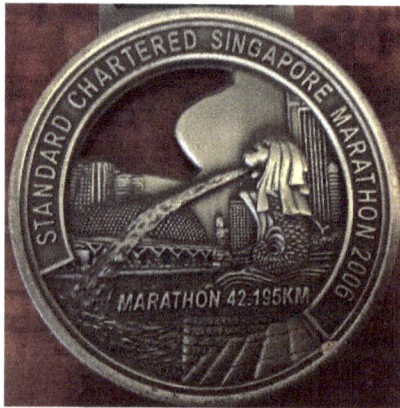

Merlion on the Singapore Marathon Medal

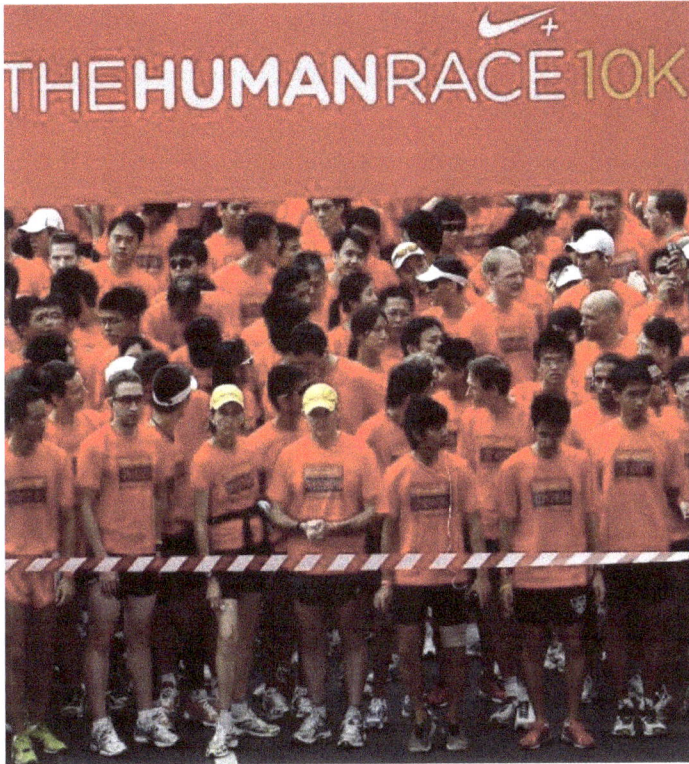

Running in Singapore (we are in the yellow caps)

Singapore has a tropical rainforest climate with no distinct seasons, uniform temperature, high humidity, and abundant rainfall. Since this tropical rainforest climate is not subject to trade winds, cyclones (hurricanes) in Singapore are very rare. The daily temperatures usually range from 25 to 35 °C (77 to 95 °F) but typically the daytime temperature is 32 °C (90 °F). It wasn't unusual for it to be 29 °C (84 °F) at 11 pm. It rains all during the year but there is a wetter monsoon season from November to January and on average the sun rises at 7.00 am and sets around 7.00 pm.

We quickly came to realise that food is very important in Singapore. It's a common greeting in the afternoon to ask, 'Have you had your lunch?' Singaporean meals are as diverse as its people with a blend of Malaysian, Chinese, Indonesian, Indian, and western influences. There are many hawker centres or food courts where individuals or families run a shop to prepare and sell meals. My favourite meal was Nasi Lemak. It's a Malay fragrant rice dish cooked in coconut milk and served with fried chicken, pine nuts, sambal, ikan bilis (small fish), and a boiled egg. It's commonly found in Malaysia, where it's considered the national dish.

So, we were moving to a place where it's very hot all the time with very high humidity as it's almost on the equator. Once we were in Singapore, we had a simple plan for running. Given the heat and humidity we would simply train all year to acclimatise and plan to run the Singapore marathon which was scheduled for the first week in December. We realised we had a lot of conditioning to do to run 42.195 kilometres (26.2 miles) safely and efficiently in that sort of climate.

The year moved swiftly by, but we fitted into a running groove in Singapore. From the beginning I decided to take up karate as well, as it was a lifelong dream to learn a martial art in Asia, and Maria continued with tennis. The karate also provided me with extra flexibility training and fitness as well as a structured process to progress through the karate learning process. It must have been quite a sight to see a 47-year-old white male sitting cross-legged in the front row of the class, full of young Asian teenagers, wearing my white Gi (uniform) and white Obi (belt). I regularly took the grading assessments to measure my progress. It also supported my view that it's good to do some cross-training to support running as the cross-training, if done well, could build up the core muscles in the body and build strength in the legs and upper body.

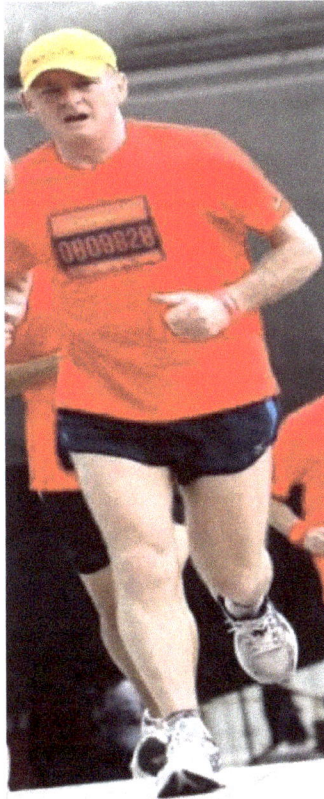

We started joining in on many of the organised running races in Singapore from ten- kilometre races to courses over multiple surfaces like roads, trails, beach sand, and hill races like the Mount Faber race. Maria really fit into a groove and in most races, won her age category and/or placed in the top three in the masters (over forty) category with prizes like free shoes, sports bags, and cash bonuses. Most runs were on flat terrain and very well supported as many Singaporeans liked to participate in running events.

Finally, the end of the year came around. We had done our marathon preparation and believed we had learned how to hydrate well in a race at 32 °C (90 °F) with high humidity. When we moved to the US a few years later most races would probably be postponed in such temperatures, but in Singapore every day was 32 °C (90 °F). The day of the race I decided to aim for a personal best of less than three hours fifty-four which was not too ambitious but given the climate I decided I would be happy with that. We decided to run our own race and from the start I set out at a nice five-minute-per-kilometre pace. Maria dropped back into the distance while I surged ahead. By halfway the heat, humidity and fatigue was starting to affect me. I was struggling to hydrate well and faltering off my pace. Five-minute kilometres drifted back to five minutes and thirty seconds per kilometre and kept sliding.

At the 35-kilometre marker, I remember it well, I

ran through a mist shower that the organisers set up to help cool down the runners. I heard some footsteps coming up behind me. As I turned around, Maria waved cheerily at me and ran on past like I was walking. This spurred me along, but I couldn't catch up. She drifted off ahead onto the finish line. As I turned down the final straight to the finish line, I realised that despite all the heat, humidity, and dehydration I would do three hours fifty-four minutes equalling my recent time at Rottnest island. Maria also did a personal best dropping her time down to three hours fifty minutes. That was marathon number four for me and number three for Maria.

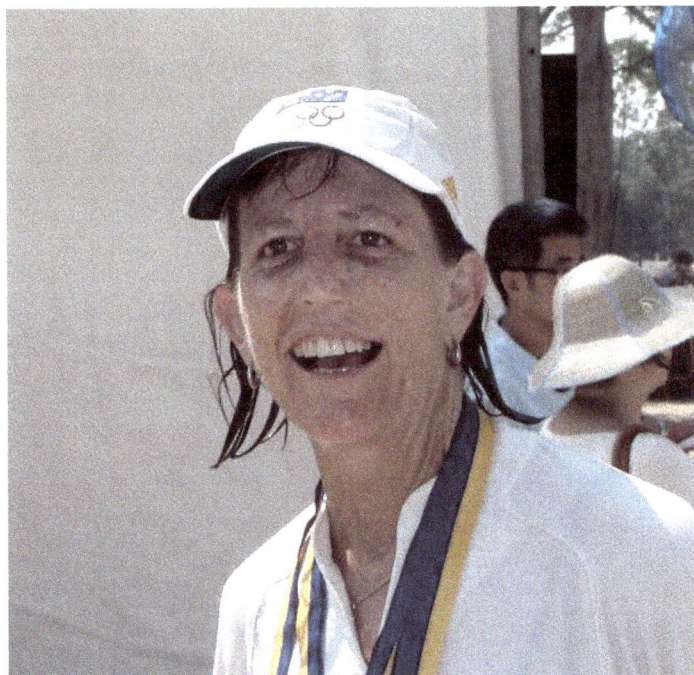

Maria — running in Singapore is a hot and sweaty business

At the finishing area we were given a cold drink, a finisher's medal, a black marathon T-shirt and something to eat. This was typical of Singapore as the whole running festival was organised amazingly well. Over our time there the race organisation would just get better and better. People were provided with shade and a free massage as well to relieve their tired muscles.

When we were walking back to collect our sports bags, I started talking with a runner who turned out to be from Germany. We chatted about the race and what races were in Germany. He was a keen if not fast runner and had completed marathons in Germany in places like Berlin, Munich, and Frankfurt. During our brief conversation he said some words that would stay with us for years to come. He said, 'On holidays, I travel, and I organise to run a marathon at my destination'. I asked what he meant by that and he added that if he was going to take a holiday in Spain he would schedule in a marathon in Spain while he was there. This holiday he was in Southeast Asia, so he scheduled in a marathon in Singapore. So, these simple words stuck in our minds. We could travel and do marathons!

As Singapore was a very central location in the world with inexpensive flights to many other locations, we could travel, take short breaks and run in many places. There were overnight flights to London, many places in Europe, Africa, and shorter flights to Southeast Asian countries, Japan, China, and Korea. Running in other countries was a small concept which would flourish into an amazing series of big adventures taking us all around the world.

> *'The question is not how many years*
> *in your life but how much life in your years.'*
> *Anonymous*

Chapter 6

The 'Classic' from Marathon

Imagine two people sitting on a small deck amongst a tropical garden dominated by a large green tree that shaded the deck. They were sitting around a small, simple, sun bleached wooden table under a large umbrella that was darkened with time and mouldy due to the humidity. It was evening. The sun had just gone down but it was still very hot and humid. Sweat sometimes tricked down their backs but they didn't notice it as that was normal. That would be Maria and me on a Sunday evening, relaxing after a busy work week and sometimes busier weekend. The white stucco apartment block rose above us and off to the left and right but for some reason our small ground-floor outdoor deck seemed to be private. Nobody walked along the narrow dirt path that meandered through the tropical garden. All the neighbours elected to remain indoors with the windows closed, curtains drawn, and the air conditioning switched on. In some ways it was our small sanctuary in an otherwise densely populated and busy city.

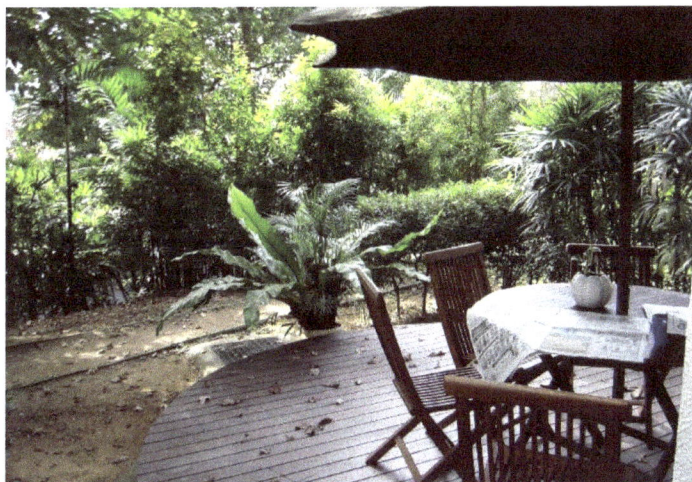

The deck, garden, and umbrella in Singapore

Maria and I were discussing what our goals and plans were for the following year. We are big believers that it's important for couples to align their goals, so they're always focused on what's important, heading in the same direction and not get sidetracked by other distractions. It was something we had learned over twenty-five years of our marriage. It worked for us. We found that once we agreed and wrote down our goals they always seemed to work out, not because they were always simple and realistic, but because we believed that the mind is an amazing thing and given time can work out how to make things happen no matter how challenging they might be.

As the Buddha is quoted back in the fifth to fourth century BC:

*'We are shaped by our thoughts;
we become what we think.'*

That year, one of the goals was to learn from that brief conversation with the German runner. It's too bad we couldn't somehow tell him that his simple sentence had such a profound impact on us and provided us with so many exciting ideas. We decided, from his comments, that when we travelled, we should use that opportunity to do a marathon. To some people that would seem absurd. Surely sitting on a beach on a tropical island sipping a margarita, reading a novel would be best or sailing off on a cruise into a beautiful island archipelago with the sun warming your face and the breeze ruffling your hair. Not running a marathon on holidays. And yet the conversation was not if we would run a marathon on holidays but where and when. It reminded me of the quote:

*'Sometimes the people around you
won't understand your journey.
They don't need to, it's not for them.'*
Anonymous.

We then googled 'marathons' and got 62 million hits. After some more thinking we googled marathon and Athens. The logic was that if we were going to travel and run marathons, we should at least start with the original marathon from the town of Marathon in Greece to Athens. But did such a run exist? After the internet search we found that it did exist, and it was marketed as the Athens Classic (authentic) Marathon. We discovered that a running festival is held in early November each year and it comprised a range of race distances. It normally attracted over 40 000 competitors, and in most years over 15 000 completed the 42.195 kilometres (26.2 miles). The race began in 1972 and is considered perhaps the most difficult of the major marathon races as the course is uphill from the 10 km mark to the 31 km mark which is the toughest uphill climb of any major marathon. The course begins in the town of Marathon, where it passes around the tomb of the Athenian soldiers, and it traces a path near the coast through Nea Makri. Then the course goes slightly downhill towards the city of Athens finishing up at the Panathinaiko Stadium which was a site for athletics competitions in ancient times and the finishing point for both the 1896 and 2004 Olympic marathons. The words 'major marathons' were new to me. I assumed they referred to the popular big races like London, New York, Berlin, Tokyo, Chicago, and Boston. These didn't really appeal to us as there would be very large crowds, but over time we would run in some of those locations.

With 'The Classic' selected, we decided to look for a race earlier in the year closer to Singapore and found the Phuket Marathon in Thailand. It was close by, and there were very low-cost budget flights from Singapore to Phuket. The Phuket Marathon is in mid-June each year and from the reviews it was well organised provided beautiful scenery. That amounted to a plan of three marathons that year. First Phuket, then Athens and finally Singapore at the end of the year. I wrote down in my goals that year the quote:

> *'Your only limitation is your imagination.'*
> — Anonymous

Singapore is an interesting place where multiple nationalities of people live in harmony. At the office, I worked with Singaporeans, Indian Singaporeans, Japanese, Chinese, Americans, Australians, Canadians, New Zealanders, English, Taiwanese, Koreans, and Malaysians. Singapore was also, on a superficial level, the land of Tiger beer, Orchard Road, beautiful orchids, a great public transport system, political stability, safety, cleanliness, the Marina, and the botanical gardens. As we lived a kilometre (0.6 miles) from the botanical gardens just off Stevens road we used to run to and through the gardens four or five times a week. The traffic is usually busy on the roads and the footpaths can be uneven and precarious. The botanical gardens however offered a peaceful and easy place to run with flat safe paths and it is much larger than many people realised. We would enter the gardens from the Nassim gate and run down through the gardens exiting either on Nassim Hill Road or the main road Napier Road. Each road delivered us back home after a nice 10-kilometre (8 mile) run.

Initially it took us a while to work out how to do the long runs on a Sunday afternoon. As it was hot all day from morning to night it didn't matter what time you went for a run. Twelve midday was just as hot and humid as 9 am, 4 pm or 6 pm. The other thing was that I sweated a lot when I ran in that environment. One time we decided to run to MacRitchie Reservoir, run the 11-kilometre MacRitchie nature trail and then catch a bus back home. The trail is beautiful as it goes through a jungle with monkeys and other wildlife plus it's around Singapore's largest reservoir. The problem was that when I got on the bus to go back home, I sweated so much that there was a large pool of sweat on the floor underneath me. Subsequently, we either caught a taxi to a starting point such as Changi village on the east coast near to the major airport and ran back or did a 30-kilometre loop such as via Bukit Timah nature reserve or out to the Singapore River through Robertson Quay, Clark Quay past the F1 track and out to the Kallang River and back.

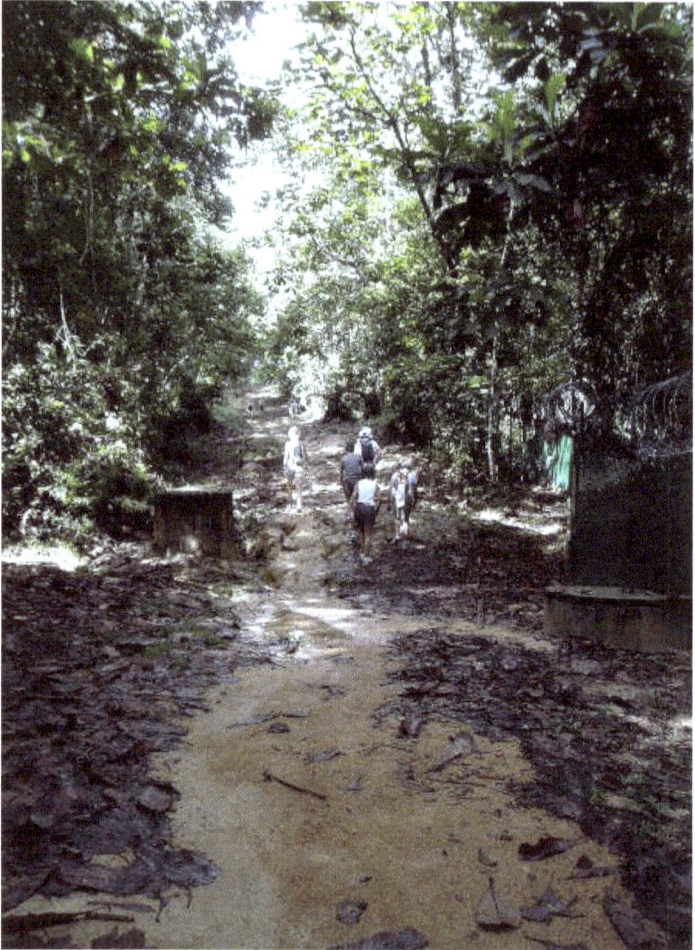

MacRitchie Nature Trail

In May that year I found out that I needed to be in the United States on business when we were scheduled to be in Phuket to run the marathon. Maria, being resourceful, decided rather than not do a run as we had done the training, she would check what were the alternatives and asked me if I could break up the return flight. I wasn't sure what she meant but finally she found a marathon in Hawaii which would be run on the weekend I was scheduled to return from the US to Singapore. Travelling east to west resulted in little jet lag for me so a stop in Hawaii was no problem and the cost was the same as a direct flight.

The marathon she had selected was on the big island and is called the Big Island International Marathon. It was also marketed as a Boston qualifier which I did not understand the meaning of at the time. The flights to Hawaii arrive on the island of Oahu at Honolulu and then it was a short flight to the Big island. The marathon was scheduled to start and finish at the Outrigger Resort near the famous town of Kailua Kona. Kailua Kona is home to the annual Kona world championship Iron Man triathlon which is a 3.86-kilometre (2.4-mile) swim in the ocean, a 180-kilometre (112-mile) road cycle followed by a 42.195-kilometre (26.2-mile) marathon race. It's widely considered to be one of the most difficult one-day sporting events in the world. It was originally held there in 1978. The trademark logo is:

*'Swim 2.4 miles! Bike 112 miles! Run 26.2 miles!
Brag for the rest of your life'.*

Maria flew into Honolulu, stayed there for a few days to acclimatise, and then flew to the Big Island. I left Los Angeles on the Friday evening and arrived at the hotel on the Big Island on Saturday in time for the run on Sunday. Travelling east means you gain time, travelling west you lose time. Sometimes this can be confusing especially with the International Date Line which is an imaginary line on the earth's surface running north to south defining the boundary between one day and the next. This line runs between Hawaii and New Zealand. Many years later Maria and I were in Auckland, New Zealand for New Year's Eve and then travelled to Hawaii on New Year's Day. We duly arrived at our hotel in Honolulu only to be advised we didn't have a booking as we were booked in from the following day. At first, we didn't understand, but it dawned on us that we left New Zealand on the morning of the first of January and arrived in Hawaii on the evening of the 31st of December. We had in fact gone back in time from one year back to the previous year! We had booked our hotel room from the first of January.

We both had an enjoyable race in Hawaii as we raced alongside historic roads with breathtaking views of the Pacific Ocean, beautiful beaches, scenic waterfalls, lush tropical forests, expansive sugarcane fields and roads through black lava fields left over from a volcanic eruption many years ago. It was humid and hot but not as oppressive as Singapore. It was also reasonably flat with some long upward areas along the route but no major hills or mountains to run up and down. As there are many Japanese in Hawaii the commentator spoke in both English and Japanese, so everyone understood his comments. I recall one lovely act of kindness during the race. At that time there was a time limit and as the time approached the announcer commented that there were still two people still out in the race. One was a 59-year-old lady from Arizona in the US and a young lad from Hawaii who was accompanying her. Remember this was then a small local marathon with 175 participants but today is billed as a big international marathon. As the marathon clock ticked closer to the time limit the race director calmly walked down to the clock and stopped it at exactly one second before the time limit so when the last two runners crossed the finish line to loud applause and cheers they were duly awarded their finisher's medal. Many years later when we were running the Two Ocean's marathon in Cape Town, South Africa, we observed a vastly different application of the cut-off time process.

The wasp

The next day after the marathon we stayed on the Big Island to relax, recover from the race, and do some sightseeing. In the morning we strolled along the beautiful beaches and went for a swim. At lunchtime we walked from the hotel along the main road and waited at a set of traffic lights to cross the road to a small shopping centre where we planned to have lunch at the local Subway restaurant. I was standing behind Maria at the traffic lights and saw a large yellow and black wasp suddenly appear and land on her neck. I found out afterwards that these yellow and black wasps are called Western Yellow Jacket wasps and are known for their aggressive nature. Before I could call out to Maria, the wasp stung her and flew off leaving her wincing in pain. Up to this point Maria had never been affected by wasp or bee stings. In the past she had been bitten by a bull ant and her foot became swollen slightly but other than that she didn't have any adverse effects from an insect sting. Bull ants are large ants in Australia that can grow up to 40 mm (1 to 2 inches), have large eyes and long, thin mandibles with a potent venom-loaded sting.

We continued our walk to get some lunch and Maria complained about the sting and rubbed her neck. At the Subway restaurant we waited to be served, collected our sandwiches, and walked outside to sit in the shade at a table and chairs setting on the patio. Maria complained again about the sting. She said she was having some trouble breathing, her face felt tight and she felt dizzy. I looked at her and her eyes, lips andcheeks were swelling alarmingly. I didn't know what to do as it looked like she was swelling up, choking, and dying in front of me! I looked around for someone to ask about the location of a doctor's clinic. I started to panic a bit as she slumped forward in her chair onto the table. Fortunately, I saw a doctor's sign just 20 metres (20 yards) away in the shopping centre. So, we abandoned our lunch. I supported Maria and made our way to the doctor's clinic where as soon as the nurse saw her, she called to the doctor and took her into the emergency room. They asked me to stay in the waiting room and mentioned something about a severe allergic reaction from the wasp sting. Maria was having an anaphylactic shock reaction which they said can be fatal.

I learned later that the doctor injected epinephrine (adrenaline) to reduce the severity of the allergic reaction and reduce inflammation in her air passages. They kept her for several hours to observe her as she recovered, and the nurse commented that she seriously considered calling 911 for an ambulance to take her to the hospital as an emergency. Maria did recover well and the doctor discussed with her that it appeared she has a severe allergy to wasps and most probably to bee stings as well so she needed to be very careful in the future and prescribed for her an EpiPen in case of a future attack. If she did get bitten by an insect, she would need to inject herself with the EpiPen. Consequently, Maria always carries an EpiPen with her. I thought about what would have happened if she were stung by a wasp in the middle of the race yesterday. She certainly wouldn't have gotten the rapid emergency treatment. Luckily that day she was very near to a doctor's clinic when we had lunch.

Next up was the marathon from Marathon in Greece. To do the travel easily, we decided to go with a Boston-based tour company. The advantages of this were that they organised all the connections from and to the airport, the accommodation and travel to the marathon start line and from the finish line. They also provided some daytrips around Greece and in Athens to see the famous landmarks like Syntagma Square, the Parliament and the Evzones, Temple of Olympian Zeus, The Acropolis, the Acropolis Museum, Areopagitou Street, Areopagus Hill, the Plaka and Monastiraki Square. We also had the opportunity to taste some delicious food in Athens like tzatziki, dolmades, moussaka, baklava, and my favourite a Greek salad with fresh tomatoes, Kalamata olives and feta cheese.

A very welcome addition to the group was that a well-known former US Olympian, marathon runner, author and running coach was joining the tour, Jeff Galloway. Jeff was a member of the 1972 US Olympic Team in the 10 000 metres and according to the legend was also famous for not winning a race. It's reported that Galloway, along with his Florida Track Club teammates Shorter and Bacheler, made the 1972 US Olympic team, Galloway in the 10-kilometre race, Bacheler in the marathon, and Shorter in both events. In the Olympic trial for the marathon Galloway reportedly paced his friend Bacheler through the race and then dropped back just before the finish so that Bacheler could take the remaining spot on the Olympic marathon team as Galloway had already qualified for the 10 000 metres. Bacheler had narrowly missed out qualifying in the 10 000 metre trials earlier.

Prior to travelling to Athens, we read Jeff Galloway's

running book and learned a lot from his experience. One key suggestion was to take short walk breaks during a marathon. The advantages, according to Jeff, were that you would run a faster race as you reduce fatigue by taking regular short walks, especially early in a race, and you break up the distance into manageable units. So, here was a former Olympian stating that it was worthwhile to walk a bit to run better. We decided this was worth trying and chatted with Jeff on this while in Athens with him. One of his main aims was to also train people who would not normally run to get off their couch and run and he was very successful at this. We decided to walk for 20 seconds through each drink station, take a drink and start the run again. This included the very first drink station.

On race day we came out into the foyer of the hotel and were confronted, for the first time, with some of the characters who run the bigger races. One man from California in the USA was standing in a replica Roman centurion's steel uniform together with a steel battle helmet, spear and shield. I had no idea how he was going to run a marathon in that uniform, but he did.

The morning at the start line was cool and fresh and the race started over the first five kilometres with the first diversion around the two tumuli or burial mounds. One is a burial mound that contains the ashes of 192 Athenians who fell during the Battle of Marathon in 490 BC. The other contains the inhumed bodies of the

Plataeans who fell during that same battle. The course is relatively flat past this point to the 10th kilometre mark (Nea Makri) and from the 11th to 17th kilometre the route goes up and down small hills before starting a steep ascent with the largest ascent at kilometre 20. The last and most difficult part of the course starts from Gerakas and goes up to Stavros Junction (30 km — 31 km). After this the route descends to the Agia Paraskevi Square, goes through the districts of Chalandri and Cholargos, and flattens out in the city centre to the finish.

The race went well, and we had decided to run together. We did the run/walk/run method and felt it was working for us. The route was predominantly within the city and town areas. The streets all along the race were lined with thousands of people cheering for the runners. They ranged from the very old to babies in arms, older ladies in dark clothing to the younger ones dressed in all shades of colour. The race was warm but not hot and while it was quoted as an upwards journey for the first part of the race, it felt manageable. Finally we rounded a corner and the magnificent, marble Olympic Panathinaiko Stadium came into view. We ran onto the stadium running track and under the finish line doing a personal best of three hours forty-four minutes. Maria had tears in her eyes. Such was the emotion of finishing this magnificent original marathon in such a magnificent setting as the ancient Olympic stadium. Both of us were exhausted.

After the race we went under a marquee to rest and

get changed out of our sweat-soaked running gear. Here we realised three more key things:

1. Taking small walk breaks through each drink station worked for us as we did personal bests on what was supposed to be the most difficult course of the major marathons.

2. The second was when another runner pointed to a female runner across the other side of the marquee and said that she had run a marathon in Antarctica. This was news to us. Can you really run a marathon in Antarctica? Apparently, you can.

3. The third was that she did it as part of becoming a member of the exclusive runners' Seven Continents Club. What was the Seven Continents Club? To join you needed to run a certified marathon on each continent.

We had already run in Australia, Asia, North America (Hawaii) and now Europe so we had already done four continents. We decided that we should set a goal to run the seven continents which left us South America, Africa, and Antarctica, on holiday of course. We were also becoming fascinated by difficult and challenging races as the Athens race was quoted as being the most challenging of the major marathons, yet we did a personal best time, and our fitness and endurance were improving. People talked about other races that were physically demanding like Antarctica, the Great Wall Marathon in China and America's Greatest Challenge

— Pikes Peak Marathon — which is a trail race up a mountain to 14 000 feet and back to the start in the Rocky Mountains of Colorado in the USA. Pikes Peak is rated as America's most extreme marathon and the second most difficult marathon in the world.

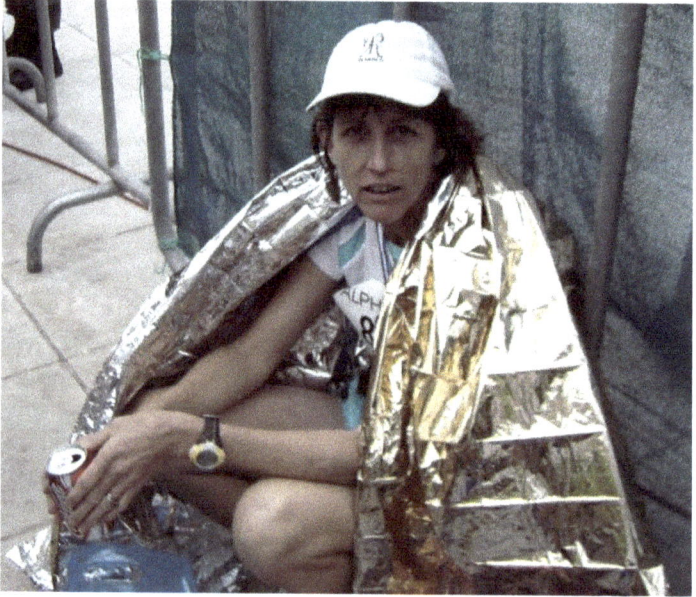

Maria — Athens marathon

'The greater danger for most of us is not that our aim is too high, and we miss it, but that it is too low, and we reach it.'
Michelangelo

Chapter 7

Running the Wall

As the year ended Maria ran the Singapore marathon on her own as I was away on business in London. The run was slower than she expected but the weather was the same, very hot and humid. Maria was also featured on the cover of Singapore's premier Health and Beauty Magazine.

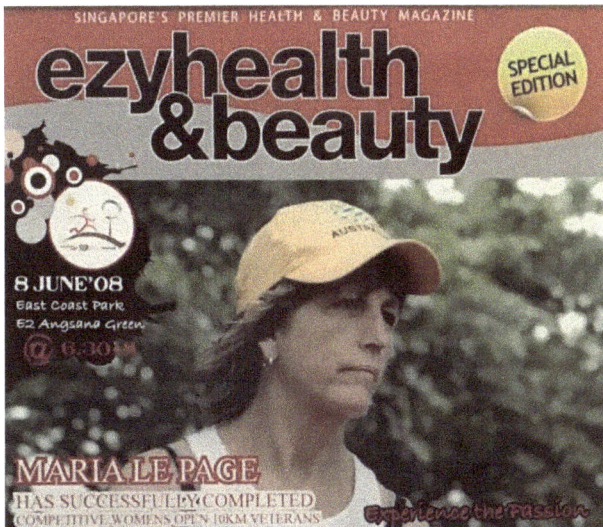

We were both now on six marathons and it was time to sit back, relax and take our time to reflect on what went well for the year and what we should do the following year. Once again, we googled and looked at the runs that were available and two immediately appealed. One was again the Singapore marathon as it was on home territory. Additionally, Singapore was planning a marathon with a twist. It was the Sundown Marathon which was scheduled to start in Changi Village on the east coast of Singapore at midnight. People would run until they finished which for some would be sunrise. It quickly became known as the Midnight Marathon. They also offered an ultramarathon where people could start the marathon at sundown and do the course twice giving a total of 84.4 kilometres (52.4 miles). That was the reason for the Sundown Marathon title.

I had never heard of the term 'ultramarathon' before and after asking some questions and doing a Google search I found that technically it was anything greater than the standard marathon distance. Normal ultramarathon distances are multiples of 50 kilometres and 50 miles, that is, 50 kilometres (31.069 miles), 100 kilometres (62.137 miles), 50 miles (80.467 kilometres), and 100 miles (160.934 kilometres).

By this time in Singapore I realised that it would still be hot and humid even at midnight when it was typically 29 degrees C (84 degrees F), so there was no real benefit with the weather but it would be interesting to do, certainly a novelty as we had never run in the middle of the night before. On reflection it was like when we climbed Mount Kilimanjaro in Tanzania many years later with our friends Jewel and Cyndy. The last climb from the base camp up the final section of the crater and along the lip of the crater to the highest point also started at around midnight. The outcome would be the same. Doing a high endurance effort, from midnight when you would normally be sleeping, is exhausting. For Singapore it was the midnight start, the heat, the humidity, and lack of sleep. For Mount Kilimanjaro it was similar, but it was cold, very cold with a blizzard at the top of the crater instead plus the lack of oxygen and altitude sickness. Even though each breath still contained 20 per cent oxygen at the summit, it's much harder to fill your lungs. As a result, every time I breathed, I could take in only about half as much air, and thus oxygen, as I would if you took the same breath at sea level.

So, we had then selected two marathons for the year so far. They were numbers seven and eight. We liked the idea of an African marathon and studied that a bit closer. The two that appealed were the Egyptian marathon in the Valley of the Queens, Luxor, and the Two Oceans Ultramarathon (56 kilometres or 35 miles) in Cape Town, South Africa on the Saturday of Easter weekend. It was called the world's most beautiful marathon and is regularly sold out and attracts 11 000 people for the ultramarathon. It's often used in South

Africa as a training run for the longer, more demanding, famous ultramarathon called Comrades. We had not been to Egypt before and there was a direct inexpensive overnight flight from Singapore to Cairo. There was also an inexpensive overnight flight to Cape Town via Johannesburg. An overnight flight appealed as we could leave Singapore on a night after work and land in our destination on the following morning.

The other alternative was The Great Wall Marathon which is held on the third Saturday of May on the Huangyaguan Pass, Tianjin section of the Great Wall of China east of Beijing. It had been held since 1999 and normally several hundred participants do the race. The internet descriptions and reviews described The Great Wall Marathon as one of the most challenging adventure marathons in the world due to the extreme course conditions. It contained 20 000 unrelenting stone steps varying in height from a few centimetres to 40 centimetres. Warnings were issued like 'runners must use extreme caution as there are sections of the racecourse where you must exit the wall and run along a trail alongside the wall to avoid extreme hazards. Runners should be physically fit and in shape as this marathon can be extremely hazardous' — Wikipedia. Years later I liked the CBS, Los Angeles, July 19, 2016 article on the five hardest marathons in the world which included the Antarctic Ice Marathon, Pikes Peak Marathon in Colorado, USA, and The Great Wall Marathon in their top five. According to them, 'The Great Wall Marathon is a race that might find more crawlers than runners.' We thought for a while and decided that The Great Wall Marathon looked like a really great challenge and we put Antarctica, Pikes Peak, Colorado, USA, the Egyptian Marathon and the Two Oceans Ultramarathon on the list of runs to do. Adding to the achievements for the Seven Continents Club membership would need to wait another year. At that time, we didn't realise how tough The Great Wall Marathon would be.

The Great Wall of China is an ancient series of walls and fortifications in northern China which total more than 20 000 kilometres or 13 000 miles in length. It is perhaps the most recognisable symbol of China. The Great Wall was originally conceived by Emperor Qin Shi Huang in the third century BC as a means of preventing incursions from barbarian nomads. However, the wall never effectively prevented invaders from entering China. Construction of the 'Wan Li Chang Cheng,' or 10 000-Li-Long Wall, was one of the most ambitious building projects ever undertaken by any civilisation. From a base of 15 to 50 feet, the Great Wall rises some 15–30 feet high and was topped by ramparts 12 feet or higher; guard towers are distributed at intervals along it.

We decided to use another running travel organisation to do the Great Wall Marathon as it required accommodation in the area near the Huangyaguan Pass section of the wall plus transport to and from the race and Beijing. This made it easy for us as we simply needed to arrange a flight to and from Beijing. The race started in a beautiful courtyard of what looked like an old military fort. The courtyard was paved with large impressive black and white pavers and the Great Wall surrounded the fort, crossed the river to the right and then wound its way up the mountain. On the left-hand side, it was built up the sides of the mountain, so the starting point was in this small pass next to a small free flowing river with mountains on each side. It was a beautiful location.

On the day before the marathon we walked part of the race route which included several kilometres on the Great Wall. It was very impressive not just by the physical size of the wall but also how it was built on the sides of mountains. The top of the wall was wide enough to drive a car on and every several hundred metres were substantial guard houses. As I looked into the distance you could still see the wall meandering up and down mountains as far as the eye could see. It was an amazing sight plus an extremely impressive construction.

On the day of the race it started well with a few kilometres up a mountain on a path. Then we climbed the Great Wall and ran along and down the Great Wall back to the starting point. At this point the race followed paths out into the countryside, up and down mountains, through ancient villages and along meandering creeks. The weather was fine and warm. Along the way several runners were handing out candy to excited children who lined the many roads and tracks along which we were running. At one point we passed an old bent lady who was wearing the common blue tunic, and on her back she carried a bundle of firewood which she must have collected in the forest. So, while the race was in progress normal life continued for many of the local people. In some way it must have been to their amusement that people would travel from all over the world to run through their village.

At around the 32-kilometre point, the race once again passed the starting parade ground. I was feeling comfortable at this point until I looked up and saw that the race path headed back up the Great Wall in what looked like a near vertical climb with stone steps of 30–40 cm in height. There were thousands of them. Quickly we started to weaken, and our legs felt heavier and heavier. Runners started to stop and crawl and stumble up the unrelenting steps.

At several points, once strong runners were sitting on the steps with heads bowed, breathing deeply and clearly exhausted. And the steps kept rising skyward. Further on was a runner sitting quietly, head bowed in exhaustion and sobbing on the steps for the effort to finish seemed too much. The words from that internet description echoed in my brain, 'The Great Wall Marathon is one of the most challenging adventure marathons due to the extreme course conditions. It contained 20,000 unrelenting stone steps varying in height from a few centimetres to

40 centimetres.' At that point, the runners were trapped. They couldn't go up as they were exhausted and going down was equally painful. The only solution was for them to take a rest, regroup and move onwards and upwards.

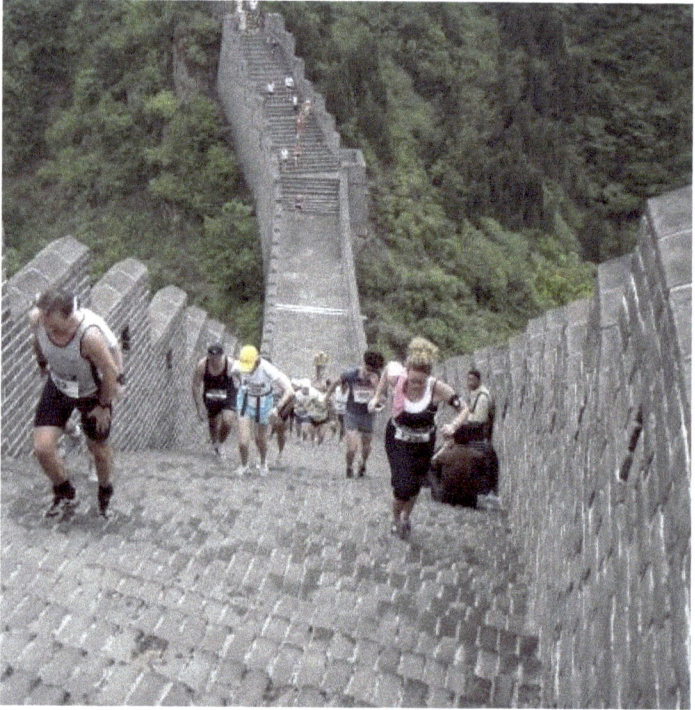

Runners during the Great Wall Marathon.
Maria is in the yellow cap

Finally, we reached the summit of the Great Wall on that mountain. The race levelled out and a five-kilometre downward run was before us to the finish line. However, I was exhausted to the point where I could barely walk. I was staggering. In marathon folklore there's a saying about 'hitting the wall' or getting to a point in the race where you're exhausted and feel you can't go any further. I had hit the wall. The Great Wall. I fumbled around in my pockets looking for some candy to eat to put some sugar back in my system, but I ended up empty-handed. I had no water either. Maria felt fine but we stayed together and after a kilometre I regained some strength and slowly ran the final kilometres down into the parade ground and finish line. We were exhausted but elated that we had finished one of the hardest marathons in the world. A cameraman came over to do an interview, but I was too exhausted to respond and politely waved him away.

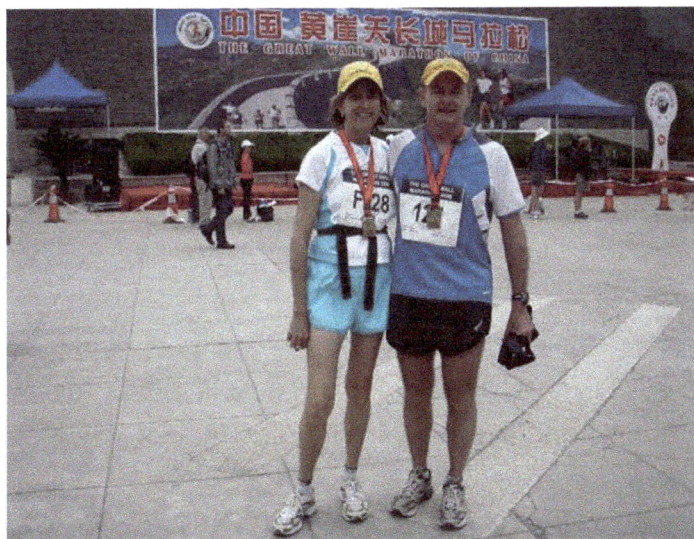

'I never would have thought one sport could change my entire outlook on life until I became a runner.'
— Anonymous

Chapter 8

Running with the Gods

The word karate is Japanese and comes from 'kara' which means empty and 'te' which means hand or arm. The word karate then means empty hand or unarmed. Other interpretations conclude that the Japanese symbol for 'kara' originally meant Chinese and void. 'Te' means hand. So, karate could also mean Chinese hand or void hand. This has led some to conclude that karate evolved from China and the practice of Kung Fu which is an ancient practice originated from the hunting and defence needs in the primitive society. The practice started in the Ryuku Islands, which are now Okinawa, Japan as the inhabitants were not permitted to have or carry weapons by the rulers. The 'do' suffix you see sometimes, e.g. 'karate-do', implies that they are not just techniques for fighting but have spiritual elements. Thus, 'karate-do' could also mean 'the way of the empty hand'. In modern times, it has developed and become not just martial skills or physical movement but also is a way of keeping fit, entertainment, and performance.

My karate black belt grading was approaching so I needed extra time to practise my katas. 'Kata' is a Japanese word meaning 'form' relating to a detailed choreographed pattern of martial arts movements designed to be practised alone and together in groups when training. It is practised in Japanese martial arts as a way to memorise and perfect the movements being executed. I had taken on the habit of while doing a training run, I would stop usually around each 2-kilometre mark to do twenty push-ups. It was a bit like cross training. Eventually I got up to 100 push-ups. It was like a university student utilising the daily commute on the bus or train as extra study time to get better.

I started practising my very complicated black belt katas while on a training run. I would do our normal 10-kilometre run through Singapore around the botanical gardens and at a set point I would stop and do a kata or two. One Sunday there were a series of exhibitions being held in the Singapore Botanic Gardens. Some were stationary and some were people performing. During this run I was stopping and practising my katas in the gardens, trying to be very precise and poised. A group of tourists gathered around me thinking I was one of the attractions. They were impressed to the point they started taking photographs and videos of me. As is the karate tradition, at the end of the long kata I stopped, stood at attention, and bowed precisely. The visitors thought that it was the end of a performance and clapped. I was not sure what to do at this point, so I smiled and bowed again.

The end of the year approached and once again we sat down to discuss our running journey and goals for the following year. It had become a lovely way of life where we did all the normal things like shop, eat, work, sleep, clean but also running was built into the weekly routine. Not running for a week would have been like not sleeping or eating for a week. It was just what we did. It also kept us very fit and energetic. At work I found I was more focused, driven to succeed and energetic, not to mention calm. My karate was also progressing. The gradings came and went and I progressed through the various belts from white to yellow to orange to blue to green to brown. At the end of the year I finally did my black belt grading which is the belt after the brown. I trained several times a week for hours at a time. The dojo (training building) was open regularly during the evening and weekends with several different trainers available so I could move my training sessions around to suit my work and other activities. At the end of the year I was awarded my black belt after a successful grading. At the ceremony, I was presented an award prepared by Ken-ei Mabuni, the Governor of the world Shitoryu Karate Association.

When Maria and I do our yearly goals, we cover a range of topics, not just which marathons we would do for the year. The topics always include a guiding statement, vision, values, family, health, leisure, investments, professional aspects (including study / training) and the plan for the year. This all fits onto one page which is stuck on the inside page of my notebook for regular reviewing to check my progress. The guiding statement is, 'I am captain of my soul. I am master of my fate. I choose how to live my life. I have a positive mental attitude and I am not disturbed by things but the view I take of them' and a secondary statement, 'If you take away a person's struggle, you take away their victory'. In case someone thinks this is all too much and they don't have the time, remember we started this a long time ago when we had four small children, and worked, studied, moved house, changed jobs and it still worked for us. Please try it.

The first statement refers to our view that we're in control of our life's journey and if it's good or bad, positive, or negative, the choice is ours. It's the view we take of it. The second statement refers to our belief that people need to make their own journey in life and be allowed to struggle, fall and get up again as through the struggle and effort they build their strength and enjoy the victories along the way. It's like an Olympic athlete. Within each athlete, without exception, is a person who has struggled, trained hard, made untold sacrifices, focused, and achieved their victory. For our running journey we knew it would take a lot of continued effort, some failures, some struggles but the journey would be worthwhile. We didn't know where it would take us, but we knew we would enjoy the journey.

> *'We are what we repeatedly do.*
> *Excellence then, is not an act but a habit.'*
> *– Aristotle*

That year we decided on three new marathons. The Seven Continent Club journey was back on the agenda, so our aim was the Egyptian Marathon to cross off Africa on the list. We also needed to be in Florida for a close friend's wedding and catch up with university friends, Dave, Jane, Sandra and Stephen so a diversion via South America on the way to Florida to do a marathon there was in the plan. Bill and Kathy's wedding was a must do event for the year in St Augustine. Bill moved to the USA nearly ten years previously, loved it and stayed. The third race was a new marathon in Perth called the City to Surf Marathon and was part of converting a 12-kilometre annual charity run from the city centre to the beach near our house into a charity running festival incorporating 4-, 12-, 21.1- and 42.2-kilometre runs. Singapore is a four-to-five-hour flight to Perth and regular low-cost flights leave on Friday evening, so it made a long weekend in Perth doing a marathon possible.

I also learnt more about the Seven Continents Club. Marathon Tours & Travel is a company set up by Tom Gilligan that specialises in travel services for runners.

It's based in Boston, USA which is the home of the world's oldest marathon — The Boston Marathon. In 1995, the company created the Antarctica Marathon and Half-Marathon. The Antarctica events enabled runners to set and reach the once unthinkable goal of finishing a marathon on all seven continents. Along with this the Seven Continents Club was formed to recognise these runners. To date in 2020, there are 527 men and 263 women worldwide who have completed this exclusive quest at the marathon distance and joined the Seven Continents Marathon Club.

Our first marathon of the year was the Egyptian marathon. After finishing a very busy week at work in Singapore and Maria also finishing a week working in her accounting business, we boarded an overnight flight to Cairo. In the morning, as our plane started to land in Cairo, I looked out over the sprawling, dusty, historical city. The sun was rising, and sunlight was spreading over the horizon providing an orange glow highlighting the ancient, famous pyramids of Giza in the distance. It was an amazing sight. I was excited to be there and was looking forward to visiting Cairo, the Sphinx, the pyramids, and the Egyptian Museum of Antiquities before running the Egyptian Marathon in the Valley of Queens near Luxor 500 kilometres (313 miles) to the south.

Cairo is the capital of Egypt and has a population of over 20 million which is the 15th largest in the world. It is located near the Nile River delta, in northern Egypt 165 kilometres (100 miles) south of the Mediterranean Sea and 120 kilometres (75 miles) west of the Gulf of Suez. The climate is hot and dry which is typical for a desert.

We booked accommodation after reading a recommendation from the Lonely Planet website. It was documented as a budget traveller's accommodation near to the museum in Cairo and was run by a gentleman who lived on the premises. When I contacted him by email, I asked if he could arrange a pickup at the airport and he confirmed he would do that. When we arrived at the airport, we were met by a lovely young man who escorted us to his car. It was a shock. The car was a very old beaten up vehicle which looked like it had been involved in numerous accidents over the years as most panels on the cars were damaged. However, he was polite, the car drove well, and we felt safe.

When we arrived at the destination, he stopped in a dusty laneway next to an old four-storey building. I asked if he was certain that this was the correct address. He pointed to the building to our right and then drove off leaving us standing there clutching our travel bags in the bright early morning sunlight. I was used to travelling on business and arriving at five-star hotels. This was a unique experience. As I looked up and down the relatively short, rubbish-strewn laneway, several old, abandoned cars littered the scene. Some cars had their doors missing and in most cases the windscreens were long gone or shattered. The cars were covered in layers of dust like the cars had been there for years. They most probably had been. On top of the car nearest to me was a large light-coloured dog sleeping in the early morning sun and another similar coloured dog was sleeping on the engine bonnet. Both dogs lifted their heads slightly, glanced in our direction and then ignored us. It was too late to ask the driver to take us somewhere else, so we went over to the building and looked at the door of the elevator. It was heavily scratched and covered in graffiti. Tentatively I pressed the up button and the doors opened revealing an inside that was as unimpressive as the outside. It was also very narrow with just enough room for two people if they stood very close together. As the elevator started rising to the top floor, I noted there was no inside door to the elevator and I could see and touch the internal walls on the building as we moved upwards. When we arrived at the top floor the door creaked open and we peered out into what looked like someone's apartment. It was nice, well furnished, clean and a pleasant voice welcomed us in. We stepped into the room and looked to the right to see an elderly well-dressed man belonging to the voice. He was standing at a small reception bench. It was indeed someone's home and he provided accommodation for travellers in four rooms.

After settling in and finding our room to be nice, well-appointed, and secure we chatted with the owner and discussed what were our plans for the day. He commented that the museum was a short walk away plus he had a friend who would drive us to the pyramids and look after us for the day for a reasonable fee. We took him up on that offer and had a wonderful day at the pyramids and in the Cairo museum. Both places were amazing and should be on everyone's list of things to see and do. I wasn't prepared for the magnificence of the pyramids nor the cluttered, amazing collection from ancient Egypt in the old museum. A real highlight was the privilege to spend time in the museum which houses the world's largest collection of Pharaonic antiquities. On the first floor there were artefacts from the final two dynasties of Egypt, including items from the tombs of the Pharaohs Thutmosis III, Thutmosis IV, Amenophis II and Hatshepsut as well as many artefacts from the Valley of the Kings and in particular the material from the intact tombs of Tutankhamun and Psusennes I. Tutankhamun's collection was particularly impressive with his jewellery, golden death mask and his chariots.

The next day we flew south to Luxor in middle Egypt which is just to the south of the ancient capital of the upper and lower kingdoms of ancient Egypt called Karnak. The Karnak Temple Complex comprises a vast mix of decayed temples, chapels, pylons, and other buildings. Construction at the complex began during the reign of Senusret I in the Middle Kingdom (around 2000–1700 BC) and continued until 305–30 BC. It's part of the monumental city of Thebes. Karnak is about 2.5 kilometres (1.6 miles) north of Luxor.

Luxor is situated on the east bank of the Nile River and from there you can see the dry, barren hills which rise inland from the west bank. It's at the base of these hills where the Valley of the Kings and Queens are, and these are the resting places of the pharaohs, the royal families, and senior members of their government.

In ancient times the Pharaoh was considered a god so as I looked across the calm blue waters of the Nile, I thought tomorrow would be a run with the ancient gods. The area around the Nile River is fertile but within a few kilometres from the river it becomes a dry, barren desert. This area in Luxor is considered to one of the hottest places on earth. Fortunately for us it was winter!

We stayed at a hotel on Kings Island. As I stared at the Nile river which is 6650 kilometres long (4130 miles) I saw small Felucca sail vessels move up and down this famous waterway and marvelled at how much rich history must have played out here over time along and around this river.

The start of the marathon was on the west bank at the entrance to the temple for a famous, female Pharaoh, Hatshepsut. She became queen of Egypt when she married her half-brother around the age of twelve. Shortly after he died, she became Pharaoh around 1473 BC. During her reign, she extended Egyptian trade and oversaw ambitious building projects including the Temple of Deir el-Bahri. She is one of the few and the most famous female Pharaohs of Egypt.

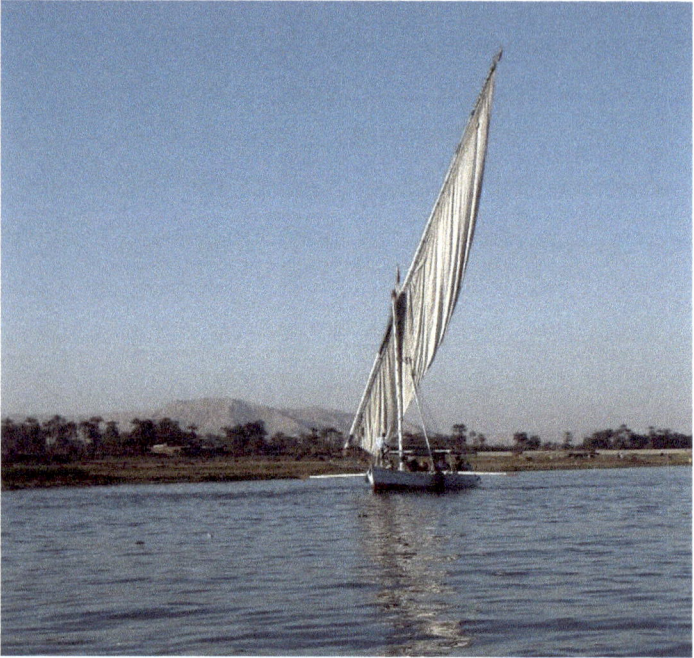

Felucca sail vessels on the Nile River

There was a strong group of runners ready for the race as the sun was rising with the air cool and still, so still that around twenty hot air balloons in a myriad of bright colours rose into the sky taking eager tourists up for an early morning view.

The 42.2-km marathon was combined with a 10-km run, the Ramses run, and a half-marathon, the Luxor run. The race took us from the base of the hills through the Valley of the Queens and down towards the Nile river. At the two-kilometres (one-mile) mark the temple of Amenphis rose to the left and two kilometres (one mile) further on the large temple to the famous pharaoh, Ramses III, rose on the right with high walls in typical ancient Egyptian architecture with hieroglyphics clearly visible. Ramses III reigned for thirty-one years between 1187–56 BC and was famous not just for the length of his reign but also because he led the defence of Egypt against invasions three times which brought peace for much of his time. He was ultimately killed in an attempted coup.

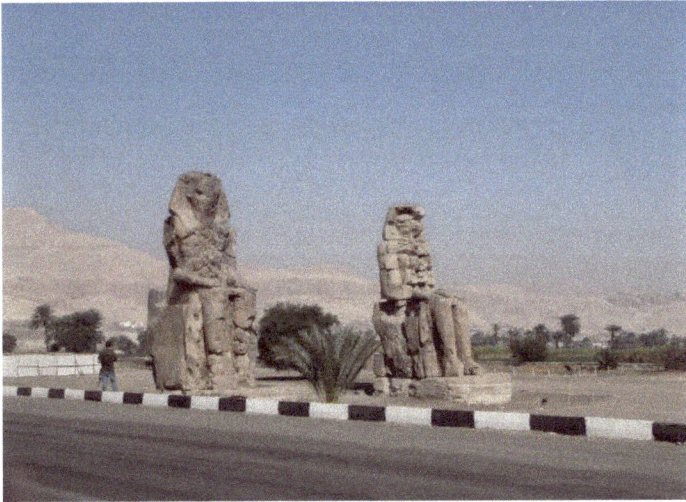

Colossi of Memnon

The air remained clear and cool but as the sun rose it became hotter and dustier. The drink stations were well-stocked and frequent. As we passed the six-kilometre mark we passed the Colossi of Memnon on the left. These are two massive stone statues of the Pharaoh Amenhotep III, who reigned in Egypt during the Eighteenth Dynasty of Egypt. Since 1350 BC, they have stood in this location and it was hard for us to imagine that these famous statues have stood in that location for over 3360 years.

One of the highlights of the run was the hundreds of local people who lined the roads cheering and offering encouragement in a language we didn't understand. In many cases a half-dozen happy excited children would run with us for 100 metres to chat and cheer us along.

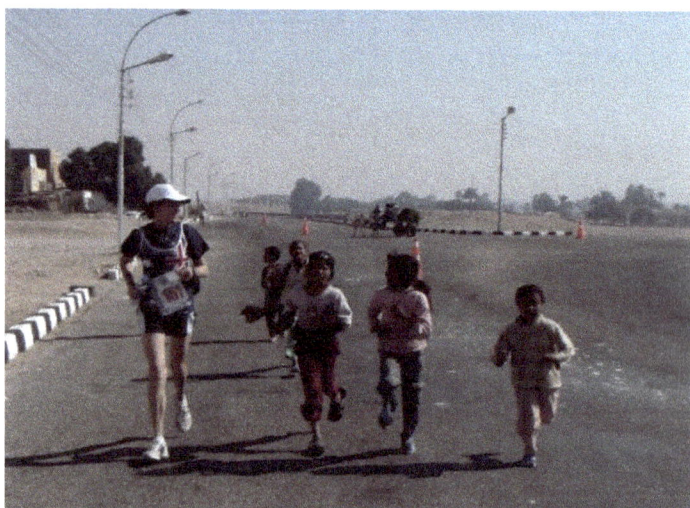

Maria running with the children — Egypt marathon

At the 36-km (22-mile) mark a white, modern station wagon passed and slowed down in front of us driving along ten metres ahead and travelling at our running speed. We thought 'Oh, what's this?' The back hatch of the vehicle slowly opened, and two people appeared. One had a TV camera, and another had a large microphone on an extension pole which they extended out to us. So, started our 'on the run' interview for the Egyptian television night-time news. We told them how exciting the run was, how privileged we were to be able to be here and run in such a historic place. It was fun for us to watch ourselves on TV that evening. The run finished back at the entrance of Hatshepsut's temple. The air was getting dustier and the tourist traffic was building for the day. The run was fun, well-organised and an amazing experience in such an ancient, famous place.

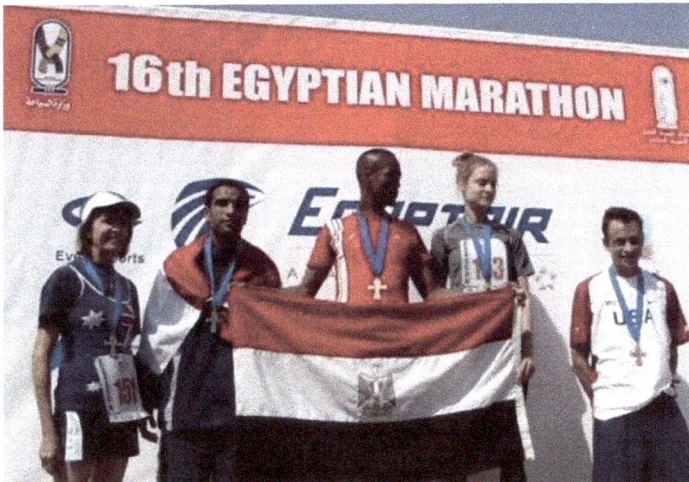

Egyptian Marathon — Maria is on the left

How did we go? We crossed the line together and ran personal best times. Maria was the second-fastest woman and was presented a silver medallion in the shape of the Egyptian hieroglyph for 'life' by the Governor of Luxor and congratulated by the Minister of Tourism. The picture is of Maria on the podium together with runners from the Egyptian Olympic male running team who collected the two top medals for the male runners. For us it was a great run and a privilege to complete it with the gods. In the evening there was a gala gathering and banquet under Bedouin canvas tents alongside the Nile River in Luxor.

Maria was one of the guests of honour as a podium finisher on the day. Here we met for the first time a runner from Pakistan, who was to become a long-term friend and fellow marathon runner. Despite the vast differences in where we lived, we would continue to meet up in four different continents for races over the next few years.

'It is important in life that for each ten years you make sure you get ten years' experience not the same one years' experience ten times.'
Arthur Le Page

Chapter 9

A PB and a BQ

Back at the finish of the Athens Marathon in Greece we heard about the Seven Continents Club for the first time along with the fact that the Boston Marathon was the longest running marathon in the world. When I did some research, I found that the Boston marathon was very popular and famous. It's run by the Boston Athletic Association which is a non-profit organisation with a mission of promoting a healthy lifestyle through sports, especially running, and established in 1887.

It's an annual marathon race hosted by several communities in the greater Boston area in eastern Massachusetts, United States. It's traditionally held on Patriots' Day, the third Monday of April, ranks as one of the world's best-known road racing events and is one of six World Marathon Majors. Its course runs from southern Middlesex County to Copley Square in Boston. The event attracts 500 000 spectators each year who line the entire 42-km (26-mile) course in rain, hail, snow, or shine. After starting with 15 participants in 1897, it now attracts an average of about 30 000 registered participants each year. In 1996 it established a record as the world's largest marathon with 38 708 entrants, 36 748 starters, and 35 868 finishers.

We liked the idea of running the world's longest running marathon and what was extra interesting was that the Boston marathon had a qualifying time to enter, often referred to in running circles simply as a BQ. This meant that you needed to be in the top ten per cent of marathon runners worldwide to qualify. The qualifying times were published, varied on age and gender, and were based upon each athlete's age on the date of the Boston Marathon. The qualifying times needed to be based on an official submitted net time (also known as chip time) from a recent certified marathon course. A chip time refers to the fact that in most marathons each runner wears an electronic chip. The chip is either built into the race number or is on a band that is wrapped around the wrist or ankle. The chip is recorded when the runner passes over the starting line and at several other locations during the race including the finishing line.

The results are then recorded electronically in a central computer system. The results are assessed to ensure each runner passed over the checkpoints along the marathon route and has run the entire distance.

Interestingly, due to field size limitations, having a qualifying standard does not guarantee entry into the event but simply the opportunity to submit for registration. In recent years, not all qualifiers who submitted an entry had been accepted. When the total amount of submissions surpassed the allotted field size for qualified athletes, those who are the fastest among the pool of applicants in their age and gender group would be accepted.

I checked our qualifying times. I needed to run around three hours 35 minutes and Maria needed to run three hours 55 minutes. For Maria each of her recent run times qualified her for Boston as she exceeded her qualifying time by 11 minutes. As we did each major race, Maria and I would run together so she was as fast as me. Regarding a BQ it was a different story for me. If I looked at my first marathon time of four hours and 4 minutes, I was 29 minutes off the pace. This meant that at that time, I would've had to beat myself by nearly 6 kilometres running at a five minute per kilometre pace. My most recent race in Egypt was three hours 44 minutes which was a personal best (PB), so I had a little way to go but I thought not bad for a 51-year-old runner. I was getting fitter and faster as I got older. Age is no excuse either.

I was still nine minutes or nearly two kilometres off the pace for a BQ time. I thought my last race in Egypt was good with a PB but a PB by seconds, not minutes, over my previous race. I needed to improve so I started on a journey of a PB each race to get fast enough to get a BQ and remembered that a qualifying time was often not good enough to get into Boston. I needed to do better than a BQ. I needed to up my training. But how?

When I scanned through some of my running books again and reread my own brief marathon training notes from several years before, I noted a couple of interesting things which I had considered important at the time but ignored either because I thought they were too hard or I simply overlooked them. They, together with one other point, stuck in my mind. The other point was a lighter runner had to have a chance to be a faster runner. After playing football my weight was around 85 kilograms or 187 pounds. When I started running a bit more, I reduced it down to 75 kilograms or 165 pounds. This was simply by eating more fruit and vegetables and less carbohydrates like bread, pasta, and rice. I have continued this since, and my weight has been stable. I decided to make a few small changes and drop two kilograms. Some of this may seem obsessive to some people, but for me it was a few simple tune-ups which could make the necessary improvements. It wasn't an overhaul but some small manageable modifications. A sailor would say it was improving the trim on the sails. A cynic would say the extra kilograms were as useful as an ashtray on a motorbike.

The other two items that I had ignored despite considering them of interest a few years ago were interval training and monitoring my heart rate. I had to remind myself:

Interval training — add in one day per week, a set of interval training during a normal run. I read a few books and they indicated that one 30-minute session was enough each week to improve fitness and speed. If more sessions were done it raised the risk of injury.

- After a 1-km warm-up sprint between two light poles, then jog for the next two light poles, then sprint between the next two light poles. Warm up 1 km, 3 km interval training, 1 km cool down.

- Another alternative is to find a nice hill of 400 metres length and after a warm-up (5 minutes), run at pace up the hill and jog or walk down — repeat for 20 minutes and 5-minute cool down.

- Another alternative is to find a football field and after a warm-up (5 minutes), run at pace around 400 m and jog the next 400 m — repeat for 20 minutes and 5-minute cool down.

- At any time, it is OK to walk as you build up your fitness.

- The aim is to do no more than 30 minutes of interval training each week so after a time the aim is to do a 500-metre warm-up and cool down with 4 km of intervals.

Consider using a *heart rate monitor* to try and maintain a heart rate at or above 140 beats per minute during each of the runs after the warm-up. The aim is to increase fitness and endurance.

While Maria was down in Perth one week, she attended a Tuesday evening interval training session with the Marathon Club of Western Australia. We had been members and ran regularly with the club on Sundays when we lived in Perth. Each Tuesday evening at 6 pm a trainer led the interval session at Perry Lakes Park. It went for around thirty minutes and involved a warm-up, a cool down, and in the middle a series of fast runs punctuated by a rest to recover after each run. The target distance was always around five kilometres. The aim was to get your heart rate into the red zone during that thirty-minute period. The red zone is 90–100 per cent of your estimated maximal heart rate (MHR). When you are in the red zone, you should feel like you are working close to your maximal effort. Your maximum heart rate can be estimated with a commonly used formula of 220 minus your age. However, research has shown that this formula is not perfectly accurate for all people, especially for people who have been fit for many years or for older people.

Some examples of typical interval training are as follows:

- 12 by 400-metre runs at maximum effort around the athletics track with a short rest in between each 400-metre run.
- Pyramid — Start with 400-metre run then increase

it to 800 then 1200 metres and then decrease by 400 metres intervals back to 400 metres.

- Pyramid — Start with 200 metres, increase to 400 metres, then 600 metres, then 800 metres, then 1000 metres, then 800 metres, then 600 metres, then 400 metres, and finally 200 metres.
- All runners start to run to 400 metres. When the first runner finishes the 400 metres the trainers blows a whistle, and all the other runners stop where they are. This point is each runner's starting point for the next fifteen runs. The trainer blows the whistle, and everyone races back to the start then rest. Repeat.
- Run 800 metres and rest. Repeat five times.
- Run 1000 metres and rest. Repeat four times — total of five

After this experience, we gathered some of our running friends in Singapore to meet each Tuesday evening at 6 pm at the National University of Singapore athletics track to do some interval training. We led the training and became running coaches. Just a few years ago we didn't know what a marathon was and now we're helping others. People would say things like 'Maria and Michael just ran a marathon in Egypt or along the Great Wall in China or in Hawaii' or 'Maria came second in the Egypt marathon.' Some would ask us questions about how to run, what did a marathon training program look like and best of all, they would start scheduling into their year a race or two to start their own running journey.

Each week we would run down to the university, meet the other runners who varied week by week as new runners joined and others departed to do the interval training and then run back home. Each week I would vary the interval training program. We often talked about the runs we did and our training. People loved hearing the stories and it was nice for us to encourage people to be healthy, to run, to train and participate.

> *'A candle loses nothing by lighting another candle.'*
> *— James Keller*

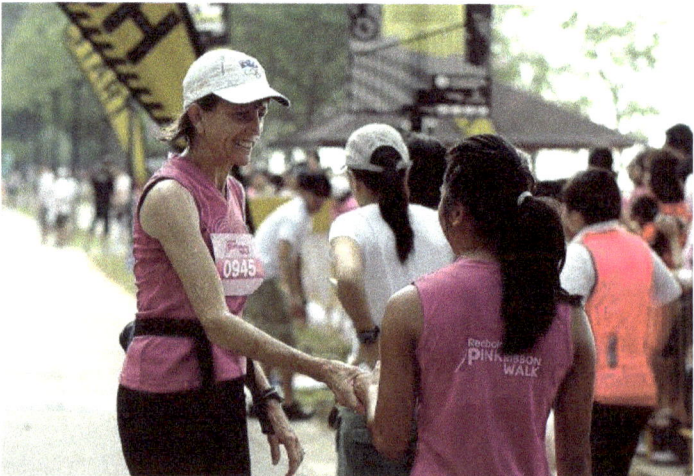

Maria — encouraging the other runners in Singapore

When the organised interval training did not occur, we would substitute that training with some hill repeat runs. We also bought a simple Polar heart rate monitor which consisted of a wristwatch and a heart rate strap which fitted around the chest.

Subsequently I have bought a Garmin heart rate monitor and currently own a Samsung smart watch. All were very good, but I preferred the Garmin with the chest strap. It was accurate and could be easily toggled during a race between speed (minutes per kilometre) and heart rate (beats per minute — bpm). I also bought a book on the use of heart rate monitors to improve performance and settled for a simple formula which was to train at least above 140 beats per minute (bpm) or more on my regular runs and try to get my heart rate over 160 bpm during the interval sessions. After some training, I would run in a marathon race averaging at 158-159 bpm and could lift it up to 170 bpm for short intervals if I wanted to overtake someone. This worked for me, but it may not work for other people, so it's best to read and try out some options for yourself. Remember to have your health checked by a doctor before starting a training program and regularly afterwards.

Over the next few months, I built the improved training into our regular routine. Prior to the next two marathons that year, we had just completed the Mount Faber race on a Sunday morning and were running back home after the race to get in some more distance. Mt Faber is not really a mountain as the height is 105 metres (310 feet) but in Singapore it's a significant landmark. During the run we dropped into a store and met a friend of Maria's called Jacqui and her husband Geoff. Geoff's first question to us was if either of us could swim. I thought this was an odd question but nevertheless responded that I could swim well. I had grown up in Australia and with the warm weather swimming was as normal to me as running. So, he asked us to form a triathlon team with him to compete in the upcoming Olympic distance triathlon event in Singapore. Geoff was a cyclist, and he was looking for a runner (Maria) and a swimmer (me) to complete his team. This was the start of our triathlon experience and more importantly Geoff subsequently introduced us to road cycling which has become a long-term passion of ours.

The Perth City to Surf Marathon was held in August. Fortunately, it was cool and calm on the morning for this inaugural event. As the runners assembled at the start, we were at the front as normal just behind the super-fast African professional runners. I was intrigued by their physique. They were typically short, thin, and lean with small tennis ball size calf muscles which is to be expected of world-class long-distance runners. When the race started, we saw them quickly drift off into the distance averaging 3.2–3.5 minutes per kilometre compared to my target of five minutes per kilometre. It was a lovely race, well organised and ended up next to City Beach. We had trimmed three minutes off our time, so it was a PB and a BQ for Maria and a PB for me, but I was still six minutes, or more than a kilometre, off a BQ time. Was I disappointed? Yes, after all that additional effort, but it was an improvement and that was what I was looking for. The BQ was in sight.

> *'Successful runners are not the ones who have never struggled. They are the ones who have never given up despite the struggles.'*
> *– Anonymous*

Later that year we headed off to Florida for the wedding via Rio De Janeiro, Brazil to complete the South American leg of our Seven Continents journey. Our journey started with a flight from Singapore to Sydney across the Pacific Ocean to Santiago and on to Rio de Janeiro. It was a long journey, probably the longest we had done to date. My reading of the marathon said the Rio de Janeiro Marathon was the largest event of its kind in Latin America and had evolved into a running festival with a variety of races. Some people call the marathon the most beautiful in the world as it starts at Recreio adjacent to the beach 42 kilometres (26 miles) to the north of the finish line. It travels along the beautiful coastline of sandy beaches, rolling clear blue surf and rugged rock formations. It passes Barra and Sao Conrado on the way to the beaches of Leblon and Ipanema before allowing the runners to travel the full length of the famous Copacabana Beach past Sugar Loaf Headland finishing at Aterro do Flamengo set against the imposing Serra do Mar Mountains. The event is quite popular with the residents of Rio de Janeiro as over 100 000 people come out to watch the race and cheer the runners on to victory.

We stayed in a comfortable hotel a few blocks back from Copacabana Beach. We had time to explore parts of Rio de Janeiro including the city centre, that famous beach, Sugar Loaf Headland, and the botanic gardens.

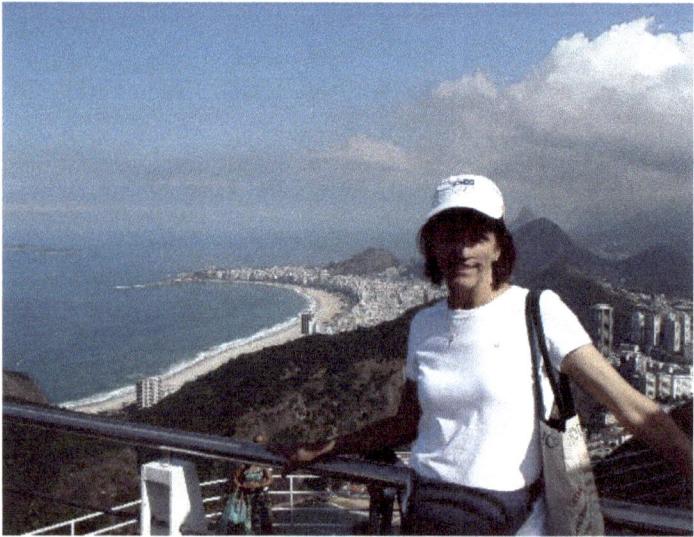

Maria with Rio de Janeiro in the background

Friends warned that Rio de Janeiro could be dangerous and for us to be careful when we were touring around. I immediately thought back to a presentation I had attended in Singapore where an airline security expert talked about travel and managing your personal safety. He had been responsible for the safety of airline staff when they were travelling especially in hotels, in transport to, from and around their accommodation. A few of his simple tips were to:

- Try and stay at reputable hotels. This doesn't necessarily mean expensive hotels. As I wrote before when we stayed in Cairo, we stayed at a place that was strongly recommended from a reputable travel / backpackers' website. It was low cost but safe, clean, and friendly plus they arranged a car to pick us up at the airport and their friend took us to the pyramids and back.

- If you have arranged for a car pickup at the airport check the identification of the driver or have a password before you put your luggage in the trunk or get in the car yourself. Once your luggage is locked in the trunk it's difficult to get it out, and once you're inside a car the inside doorhandle can be deactivated. In other words, you can be locked inside the car.

- If you need to get a lift from the airport to the hotel use a registered taxi or catch a registered bus but not someone who approaches you offering a lift for a fee.

- Keep the hotel room door open when you first arrive at your room so you can check the room to see that it's safe and empty. The open door allows you to exit quickly if required.

- Ensure the clerk at the check-in does not state aloud your name and room number together.

- Check that all the windows in your room are locked and not just closed.
- Lock the doors at night. Use the deadlock or safety chain if one is available.
- Ensure you have a torch next to your bed at night in case there's a fire and you need to exit in the dark. In remote China we did have a blackout at the hotel.
- Count the doors from your room to the fire exit so you know how to get to the fire exit in an emergency.
- When you go out walking don't take any baggage, handbags, especially expensive handbags, or cameras. These are commonly targeted by thieves.
- Do not walk alone in areas in which you don't feel comfortable. Walk in groups if possible.

Later, when we visited Cape Town, the hotel staff simply said we shouldn't go outside after dark as it was a much higher risk. Furthermore, a work colleague of mine woke up to find an intruder in his hotel room in the middle of the night. The intruder entered through an unlocked window. This occurred in Perth, Australia so travellers need to be aware at all times and in all places. The lesson is to check that all the windows and doors are locked.

On the day of the race we travelled by bus to the starting line north of Rio de Janeiro in pre-dawn darkness. Thousands of people gathered restlessly around the starting line stretching their legs, doing squats, and trying to find the rest rooms for that last-minute comfort break.

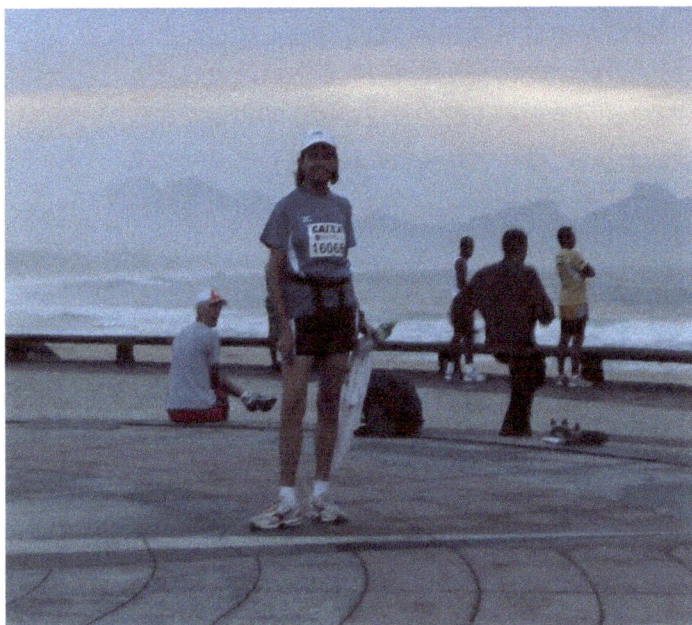

Maria at the early morning start of the Rio de Janeiro marathon

At dawn, the run started. The group of runners surged forward eager to get on their way. Maria and I decided to run our own race individually. I felt fit and well and started at a good pace. The weather was clear, still, and hot. The Brazilians that I ran with were very fit and strong. I quickly found I was running too fast as I tried to keep up with the flow rather than run my own race. Consequently, as we entered the start of Copacabana Beach my pace had slowed, I was sweating a lot and when I finished, I was exhausted and struggling on my feet. My time was up compared to the previous race and Maria came in after me. She was also exhausted and drained.

You would think that after training and running marathons in Singapore with the heat and humidity that it would have prepared us better. I wanted to lie down on the grass near the finish line and pass out, but I thought if I did that they would bring in an ambulance and take me away to a hospital so I kept on my feet looking for a chair and some shade to hide in. Maybe it was the travel or jetlag. Still, we finished the race in good time and were elated the sixth leg of our seven continent journey was complete. That left only the Antarctic Marathon to complete.

> *'Our greatest glory is not falling,*
> *but in rising every time we fall.'*
> *– Confucius*

To finish off our races for the year we decided to go to Cambodia in December to visit the famous Angkor Wat temple complex. In December there is the Angkor Wat half- marathon which is a charity event to raise money and awareness for the landmine victims in Cambodia. Angkor Wat is often listed as a wonder of the world. The list typically includes the Pyramids at Giza (Egypt), the Roman Colosseum (Italy), the Taj Mahal (India), Machu Picchu (Peru), Petra (Jordan), Chichén Itzá (Mexico), The Great Wall of China, Stonehenge (England) and Angkor Wat (Cambodia).

It's considered to be the largest religious monument in

the world, on a site measuring 1.6 square kilometres or 0.7 square miles. It was constructed as a Hindu temple for the Khmer Empire, but was transformed into a Buddhist temple towards the end of the 12th century. The Khmer Empire existed in Southeast Asia between 800 AD and 1400. Angkor Wat has become a symbol of Cambodia, and is on its national flag. The temple is surrounded by a moat which is more than 5 kilometres (3 miles) long and has an outer wall 3.6 kilometres (2.2 miles) long. I asked our guide how the moat was built, and he replied that it was dug by hand during the 12th century. I looked at this beautiful and complex temple which is in the middle of a jungle in the middle of Cambodia and marvelled at how anyone could build something so big, so amazing, and so remote so many years ago.

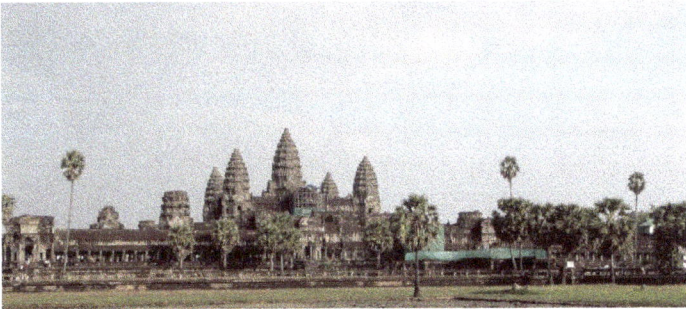

Angkor Wat Temple Complex

Angkor Wat lies 5.5 kilometres (3.4 miles) north of the modern town of Siem Reap. A few kilometres north of the entrance to Angkor Wat is the very impressive Angkor Thum. Angkor Thum literally means 'Great City' and it was the last capital city of the Khmer Empire. Like Angkor Wat it was built around the 12th century and is on the west bank of the Siem Reap River. The famous Bayon temple with its many sculptures is in Angkor Thum.

The race started just outside Angkor Wat and the route went around the outside of temple complex through the countryside and villages, past Ta Prohm Temple, and Angkor Thom, the 'Great City'. Near the end the route passed by the famous Bayon Temple and back to the finish in front of Angkor Wat. The highlight of the run was not just the amazing location and temple complexes but the thousands of local people who lined to course the cheer all the participants along.

Chapter 10

Two Oceans

Dave Venter worked for British Petroleum — Southern Africa in the 1960s and ran his first Comrades Marathon in 1967. Not long after that he was transferred to Cape Town from Durban and joined the Celtic Harriers Club which is now one of the oldest running clubs in the Western Cape based in Cape Town. It's famous for its green and white hooped running shirt. The Comrades Marathon he ran was first run in May 1921 with 34 starting participants of whom only 16 finished. As explained previously, the race is now run between Durban and Pietermaritzburg in KwaZulu-Natal Province and the direction of the race alternates each year between the 87-km up run (starting in Durban) and the 90-km down run (starting in Pietermaritzburg) with a current cut off time twelve hours. Typically, twenty per cent of the runners do not finish within the cut-off time. The race was the idea of World War I veteran Vic Chapman who wanted the race to be a lasting memorial and unique test of the physical endurance of the entrants. Today it is the world's largest and oldest ultramarathon.

When Dave Venter moved to Cape Town, he was reportedly disappointed that there were only a few marathons and no ultramarathons run in the city in which he could train for the Comrades race. So, he went on to convince his running club and the then Western Province Amateur Athletics Association to allow him to organise the Cape's first ultramarathon (56 km / 35 mile) race in May 1970. He promoted it as a training run for Cape Town athletes preparing for the Comrades ultramarathon. The race entry fee in 1970 was 50 cents and it attracted 26 runners. Recently the event attracted foreign runners from 84 different countries and, including South African runners, there are now typically 11 000 participants. The fees have increased as have the number of participants. For an international runner, the cost is now A\$170 / US\$123. Local runners receive a lower entry cost of A\$47 / US\$34. The Two Oceans Marathon was now in our plans for the year.

The year was also planned to be our last year in Singapore. We moved to Singapore to stay three years, but it rolled into four years and this year would be five. I really enjoyed living in Singapore. This wonderful, small city country, although densely populated, was clean, safe, and very well organised. My work was very multicultural, exciting, demanding, and diverse but as the old saying goes 'all good things must come to an end' which is a wise reminder that all good things are temporary. We decided to move back to Australia at the end of the year. This meant we would have one more year to book an inexpensive flight away.

After completing the South American leg of the Seven Continents journey it just left us with the Antarctica Marathon to complete so we made contact with Marathon Tours and Travel in Boston only to find out that the race was fully booked for the following year and the year after that. We then needed to put ourselves on a wait list which we did. The race is held every year in late February or early March as this was the time the ice sheet retracted back enough to allow people like us to land on Antarctica safely. Even at this time it can be treacherous. One year the runners couldn't reach land to run the race as the weather was so unfavourable. In the morning of the planned marathon there were forty-mile-per-hour winds and six-foot-high waves. The ship's captain said it was too dangerous to land the Zodiacs. This was in 2001 on the Russian vessel named the *Lyubov Orlova*. The tour organiser Thom Gilligan devised a plan that the runners could run the entire marathon in Antarctic territory but around the deck of the vessel. He calculated it would take a total of 422 laps of the deck. Over 24 hours while running in three shifts of afternoon, midnight, and the following morning 108 runners completed the marathon distance around the ship. As you can imagine running around a vessel in rough seas there were more than a few injuries with runners bumping into each other and the steel structures of the ship. However, the runners were elated as they had come to Antarctica and run a marathon. It also earned a place in running history as the first organised marathon run entirely on a ship.

The marathon is held on King George Island, one of the largest Antarctic Islands just off the Antarctic Peninsula. The start and finish is at Bellingshausen Station (the Russian base), and the course passes the Artigas Base (Uruguayan), the Frei Base (Chilean) and the Great Wall Base (Chinese). The course follows an icy track that connects the bases and changes each year based on base operations as well as the track and weather conditions.

The entire trip takes around ten days and leaves from the southern port at the tip of Argentina called Ushuaia. Normally the company contracts another company called One Ocean to charter a Russian research vessel which is set up for travel into Antarctica with the appropriate communications, sea worthiness, medical, accommodation and catering facilities. One Ocean leases various ships but the ones selected are built for polar scientific expeditions and well equipped for rough seas.

Every day once the vessel got to the Antarctic the crew would arrange transport to various points along the coast in Zodiacs (small rubber transport vessels) to cruise along and see icebergs or make landfall to see wildlife like penguins, leopard seals, various bird life and other seals. However, that adventure would need to wait for another time.

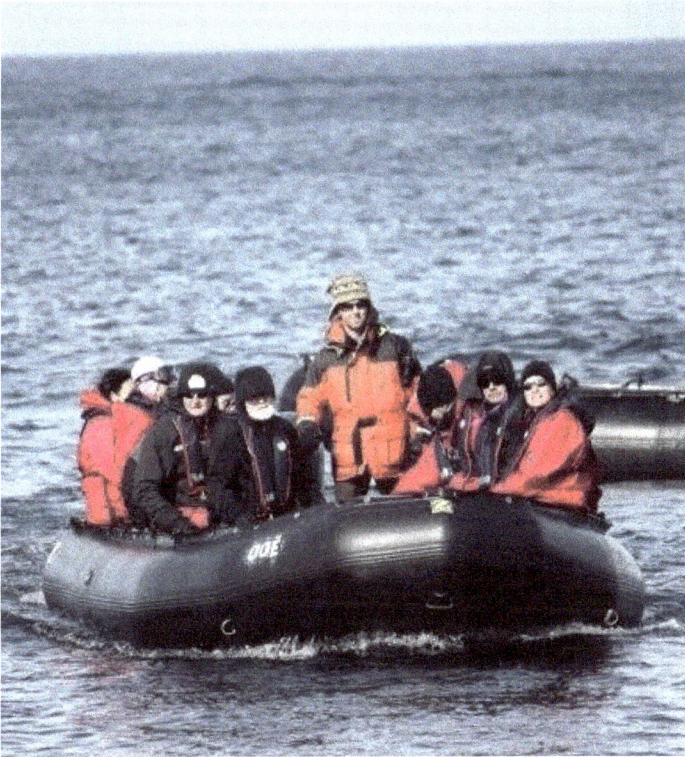

Antarctica Marathon — Zodiac transfers

After some discussion we decided on three marathons for the year. The first would be the Two Oceans Ultramarathon in Cape Town, South Africa initiated by Dave Venter. We had not run an ultramarathon before, and this race was 56 kilometres (35 miles). The second would be the Perth City to Surf again and the last one in Singapore would be the Singapore marathon.

I had never really conquered a marathon in Singapore

even though I had finished three so far. Two were the Singapore Marathon and one was the Sundown Marathon at midnight. During each I felt I had underperformed. The second Singapore marathon left me struggling down the final 100 metres of the race, very dehydrated and exhausted. I had run too fast, drank too little water, and needed more electrolytes. I finished but I laid down on the grass in the recovery area with full body cramps slowly sipping a Coca-Cola and water to put some sugar and fluid into my system. Initially I couldn't walk. I recovered but when I got home, I weighed four kilograms (nine pounds) less than normal. That was not a healthy state to be in. I was lucky I didn't end up in an ambulance on an intravenous saline drip. I learnt it was critical to continually drink water during the race and eat something with electrolytes every thirty minutes. Despite this, the weather in Singapore for a marathon is challenging. Remember, it's typically is 32 degrees Celsius (90 degrees Fahrenheit) and over 90 per cent humidity during the race. At the end of the race you typically look like you have been standing in a shower. So, for my final year I wanted to get everything right which meant to conquer the race, to finish with a personal best time for the race, feeling elated and energised.

In the previous year we had started road cycling on the weekend with our friends Geoff and Jacqui and the small cycling group called the Gerbils. Early, every Saturday and Sunday morning, we would gather at the junction of Orchard Road and Orange Grove Road in Singapore. The place is affectionately called Rats Corner. We would then either ride out to Changi near the airport along the East Coast and return or we would ride a loop through Kranji and return. The total rides were approximately 60 kilometres each and I thought it was helping with our fitness but irrespectively it was just fun to do with a nice group of people. Some of our fellow riders thought it strange for us to do the ride in the morning on a Sunday then do a 30-kilometre run in the afternoon but that's what we did.

The first marathon for the year would be the Two Oceans Marathon at Easter time. It's reported to be Africa's biggest annual running event and has earned a reputation as the world's most beautiful marathon as it takes a route around the coastline where the Indian and Atlantic oceans meet. The marathon starts at 6.40 am at Main Road corner and Dean Street in the suburb of Newlands and ends on the side of Table Mountain in the Cape Town University campus. The race at that time had a cut-off time of seven hours which was stringently adhered to. People who didn't complete it in that time didn't get the recognition as a Two Oceans Marathon finisher nor a finishers' medal.

We had arranged for a spare day prior to the race so we decided to hire a car with a driver and do some sightseeing around Cape Town and the Western Cape area. It is indeed a beautiful area and over the years I had read extensively on the history of the area and enjoyed seeing the famous Table Mountain for the first time. We drove along the proposed marathon route and it was indeed scenic. Next we travelled out to the vineyards and stopped in Stellenbosch which is a town located about 50 kilometres (31 miles) east of Cape Town, along the banks of the Eerste River. It's the second oldest European settlement in the area after Cape Town and is now home to the well- established Stellenbosch University. After Stellenbosch we drove to Franschhoek and had lunch. Franschhoek is a lovely small town of 15 000 people. The original inhabitants were the Khoisan peoples and in 1688, French Huguenot (French Protestant) refugees moved into the valley starting farms and businesses using their experience in agriculture. The name of the area changed to le Coin Français ('the French Corner'), and later to Franschhoek which is Dutch for 'French Corner'.

The following morning the race commenced in the pre-dawn and like in Rio de Janeiro, there were thousands of nervous runners milling around in the dark waiting for the start. Once that starter's gun went off, the runners headed off towards the coast in what appeared to be a southerly direction. I was immediately greeted by fellow runners using my name and asking where I was from. I then realised that my running bib not only held my name but also that I was a foreign runner. The runners were very friendly and helpful. It's not unusual for runners to chat while they run, and in Cape Town it was no different. The race was flat at almost sea level on the way down to the Indian Ocean at Muizenberg Beach. Then it followed the coastline past St James Beach and Kalk Bay which is a small bay inside the larger bay called False Bay. We went past Clovelly Beach where the route followed the coastline to Fish Hoek Beach and Faka Bay.

We were running well at a nice pace. We were well-prepared and given that the race was reasonably flat with nice scenery, particularly the beautiful coastline, it was a run that was enjoyable to this point. After Fish Hoek the path went inland, rising in altitude gradually above the scenic Noordhoek Beach and onto Chapman's Peak at around 150 metres in altitude. The route then followed the coastline again which had changed from sandy beaches to a rugged mountainous escarpment. Gradually the path descended to near sea level at the 40-kilometre mark as it went past Hout Bay and Hout Beach which was once again beautiful with white sand and blue water.

At very regular points there were aid stations and refreshments and here an unusual event happened which I had never seen before and haven't since. A crew of volunteers were serving out hot potatoes which were steaming and covered in salt. After running for several hours, sweating profusely but still in good shape and at a good pace, the potatoes and salt were not only welcome but delicious as well. Just past the 42-kilometres (26-mile) mark where a normal marathon would end, I looked ahead and saw the route steer dramatically upward to Table Mountain. The path rose steeply here by 250 metres in altitude over the next few kilometres which may not seem like a lot but after running 42 kilometres (26 miles) it was a steep climb. Finally, we reached the top at Constantia Nek. The route levelled out and started a slow decline. At the top people were giving out Mars bars or a similar sticky, sugary treat but after the past few kilometres I was exhausted and just wanted water.

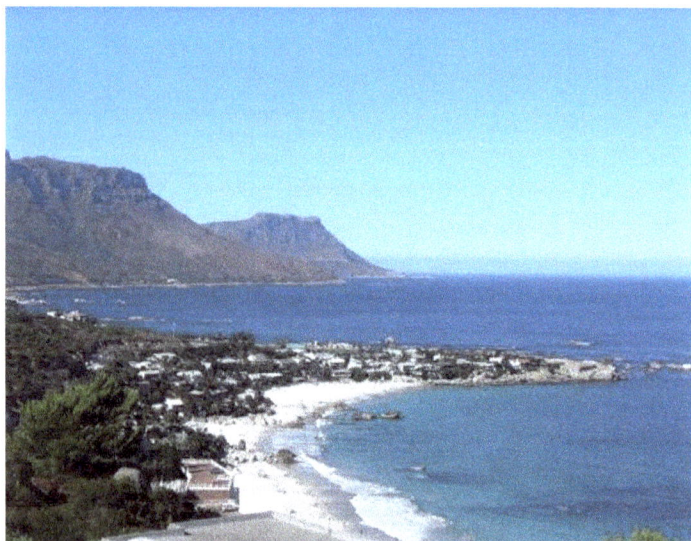

Two Oceans — coastline

From here the race went through Newlands Forest, past the beautiful Kirstenbosch Gardens along the side of Table Mountain before winding its way onto the grounds of Cape Town University. At the final turn we rounded onto the grassy section of the athletics track for the final 100 metres to the finish line and collected our finishers' medal and a cool refreshing drink. After that we rested a bit. We started to look around for another Australian who we knew was in the race that day. He was on a journey that year to complete 52 marathons in 52 weeks over 42 countries. We did manage to track him down. He was a wonderful, interesting character who gave up his career, stored or sold his possessions and went off to complete this unique challenge. Initially he had a friend with him but for the most part he was on his own.

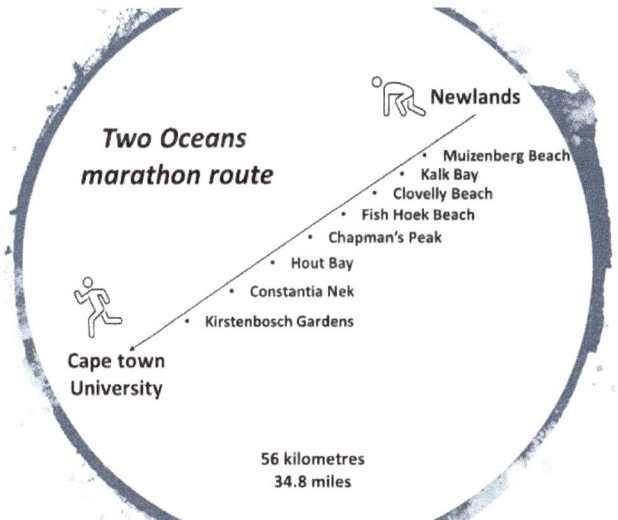

Two Oceans Marathon route

The Two Oceans Marathon was marathon 15 in his 52-marathon journey, and he had also just recently completed the Egyptian marathon, so we had a lot to chat about. He did finish his quest ending the journey with his friends completing a final and 52nd marathon in Melbourne on the 27th of December that year. After all the setbacks, injuries, the freezing cold (Antarctica), the very hot (Egypt), the loneliness, sleeping in railway stations and airports and the ultramarathons he did complete his challenge and wrote a book which he signed and sent to us. We still have a copy in our library.

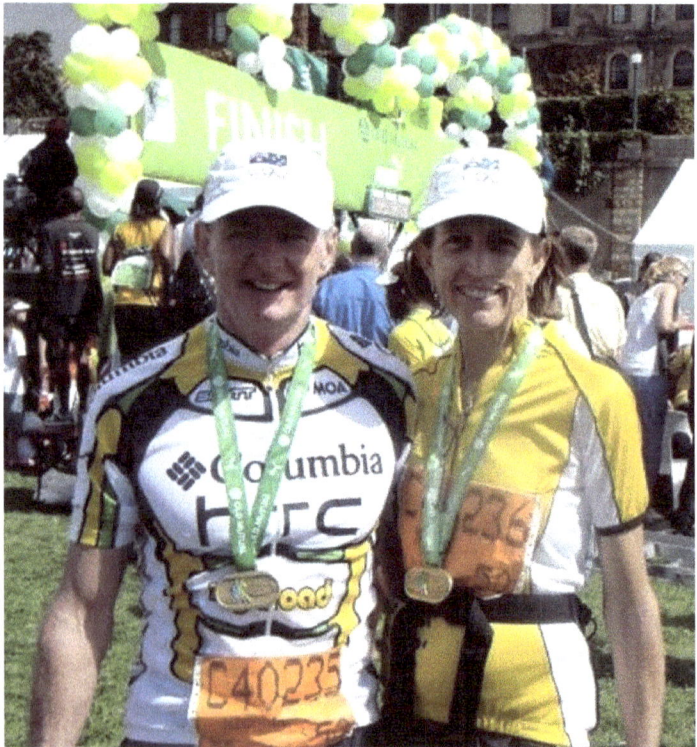

Michael and Maria — Two Oceans Ultramarathon
— Cape Town

While chatting with our new friend, the cut-off

approached for the Two Oceans Marathon. We had finished in just over five hours but there were still very many runners out on the course and some coming into the final 100 metres as the cut-off approached. As runners came around the corner you could see their eyes firmly focused on the large digital clock above the finish line. For some reason Maria, Tristan and I were transfixed watching this event unfold.

For many there was the elation of seeing the clock with enough time to run the 100 metres before the race closed. As time moved into the last minute the elation in their eyes turns to anguish or fear as they dragged their exhausted bodies over the last 100 metres. With 30 seconds remaining, there were still runners streaming onto the track racing the clock. I clearly remember one exhausted dark-haired lady race around the corner and when she saw the clock she started sprinting. Remember, she had just run 56 kilometres (35 miles) in demanding conditions involving steep climbs and hot temperatures. In her haste she tripped and fell face first into the turf. Still the clock ticked on. She looked up at the clock from the prone position, crawled, then scrambled to her feet and once again started sprinting with her focus totally on the clock like a 100-metre sprinter in the Olympics. For her you could see the race was as important as any Olympic race. You could see tears in her eyes and the strain on her face as she threw all her last energy into the final few metres to just fall over the line exhausted, crying and with just one second to spare. An official gently helped her up, placed a finishers' medal around her neck and hugged her as she wept uncontrollably.

For many of the other runners racing around that bend into the final 100 metres there was no fairytale ending, just sadness and a slow exhausted jog down the track to the now closed finish line, a nice cold drink but no medal and no official record of the finishing the gruelling race.

After the race we started to walk slowly back to our hotel along Rhodes Drive. We had been invited by our friend and some fellow runners to go to a local hotel for a celebration and a beer. As we slowly walked down the road a car pulled over and a lovely guy asked us where we were going. He said he could see we had just finished the race and looked tired. He gave us a lift back to our hotel. We were very thankful for his generosity as we were exhausted. Later that day we visited the hotel and then went to another bar in Newlands which was full of friendly people from Cape Town who joked with us and shared a drink. I was wearing a Two Oceans finishers' shirt which proudly displayed the 56 kilometres on the front. One friendly guy joked about who I borrowed the T-shirt from.

The following morning, after the race we decided to venture into the historic Cape Town port area. As we were in Newlands, we decided to walk from the hotel to the railway station, which was nearby, and catch a train into the port and return. As we walked to the train station, we passed a small side street that was lined with modern multistorey office blocks. Down the side street we saw a dead body lying in the middle of the road. Blood was pooled around the body and it looked like a well-dressed man had fallen out of one of the windows above. Did he fall or was he pushed? We didn't know what to do but after a few seconds we tentatively started walking down the side street only to see several police cars arrive and block off both ends of the street. I looked in the newspaper the next day to see if the death was reported but I never found out what happened. After that event we were even more cautious about our safety but the trip to the railway station, train ride to and from the port area were thankfully uneventful.

The following weekend we had scheduled to do an Olympic distance triathlon as a warm-up event for a 70-mile Ironman triathlon in Perth in May. The Olympic Distance, or Standard Distance, triathlon consists of a 1.5-km (0.9-mile) swim, 40-km (24.9-mile) bike, and 10-km (6.2-mile) run. The 70-mile Ironman triathlon is called an Ironman 70.3 and consists of 1.9-km (1.2-mile) swim, 90-km (56-mile) bike, and 21.1-km (13.1-mile) run. We had been cycling twice on the weekends, so we had that part and the run covered. As we both grew up swimming like most children in Australia it was easy work to prepare for the swim as well.

Initially we had booked both the ultramarathon in Cape Town and the Olympic distance triathlon in

Singapore separately without checking our calendars. It wasn't until later that I realised that we had less than one week's break between the two events. However, the triathlon went well, and we finished in good time with some of our friends from the cycling group. It was interesting that the winner of the lady's section was from England and the previous year when she did the race, she finished poorly compared to her standards due to the extreme heat and humidity in Singapore. Her response was amazing. Back in England she installed a running treadmill and a stationary road bike inside a sauna so she could set the temperature to 32 degrees Celsius and humidity 85 per cent to match Singapore conditions and train! How did she go? Well she won of course! What an amazing and determined lady she was. She reminded me of the quote.

'Life is like a camera. Just focus on what is important.
Capture the good times. Develop from the negatives.
And if things do not work out just take another shot.'
— Anonymous

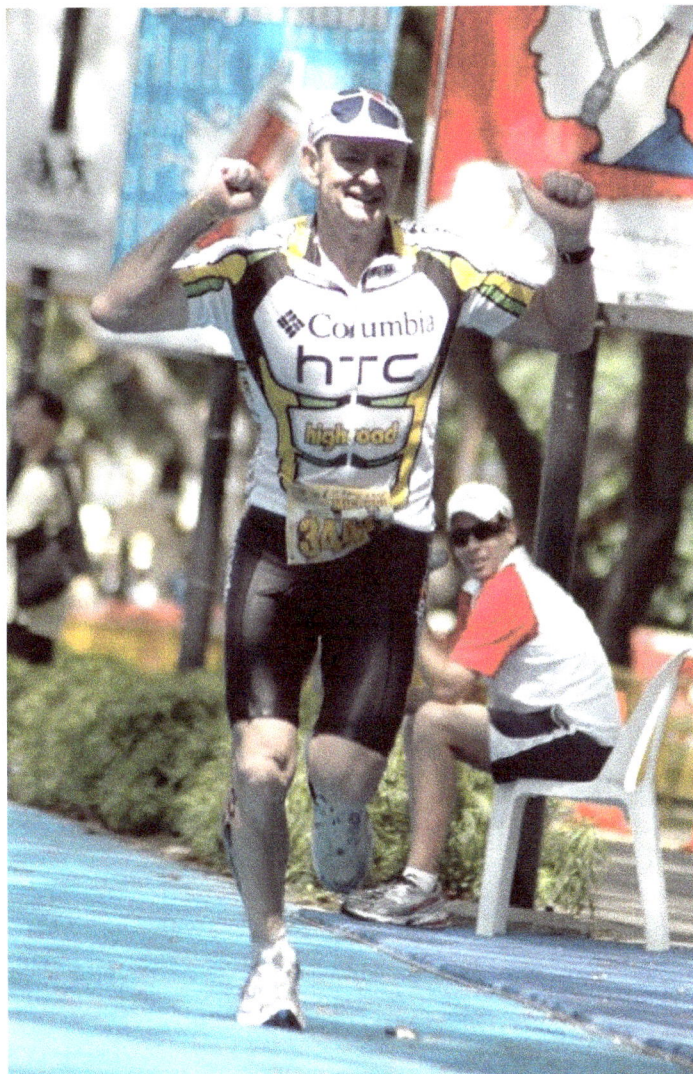

Michael — Singapore Olympic distance triathlon

After a busy April and May we went back to our normal routines. The next marathon on our schedule was the Perth City to Surf in August. We started to ramp up the training through June and when the time came to fly down to Perth. We were fit, healthy and looking forward to the race. As Singapore is hot and humid all the time I stopped trying to go for a run early in the morning or late in the afternoon on weekends as it was always hot so I would go for a run when I had time. On a Sunday, if I had time at midday or 1 pm, I would go for a run as it didn't make any difference.

I found cycling on the weekends very enjoyable as they were a nice group of friends plus cyclists like runners are interesting people. If a cyclist goes away for a weekend it can mean doing at least two long rides. So, the group in Singapore would travel over to Desaru in Southern Malaysia on a Friday evening after work, complete a 100-km ride on the Saturday, follow it up with another long ride on Sunday, travel back to Singapore later in the afternoon and go back to work on Monday. That's normal for a cyclist. Sometimes it would reach 40 degrees Celsius (104 degrees Fahrenheit) in Malaysia, but we still rode. I think this helped the running as well.

As I had mentioned previously, I often ran regular routes in cities when I travelled. We also developed the habit of going for runs when we were on holiday to keep up our training program. It's a wonderful thing to visit another place and run through the streets and parks seeing all the sites. During this time that year we went on a week's holiday in Rome. I had been in London on business and after an exhausting work period we decided to take a week off and Maria meet me in Rome. We selected a small hotel just a few streets down from the railway terminal as we caught the train into the city from the airport. Initially we walked around the city to see the various famous landmarks, like the Vatican, Julius Caesar's statue, the Colosseum, the River Tiber, the Spanish Steps, Trevi Fountain, and the many wonderful Piazzas. Once I worked out the layout of the city, we went for a run each morning. Typically, we would run from the hotel over to and up the Spanish Steps to the Villa Borghese gardens, through the gardens and down to the River Tiber across the bridge and down to Vatican. I really enjoyed running to and around the Vatican as it's such a historical place and to have the freedom to run around Saint Peter's Square in the early morning without the crowds is a real privilege. We would then run down beside the river to the Ponte Garibaldi then over to and around the Colosseum before running past Caesar's statue and back to the hotel for breakfast. It was a lovely way to start the day and like my dad many years before we felt energised and ready for the day.

Up to this point I hadn't completed a PB and BQ in any race. Maria had done it many times but with the triathlon training and the weekly interval training I had positive ambitions about this City to Surf marathon. This was especially the case as it was winter in Perth at that time so it would be cool at the start at around 10 degrees Celsius (50 degrees

Fahrenheit) and would reach 18-20 degrees Celsius (64-68 degrees Fahrenheit) during the race. That would be ideal conditions for running in Perth. Race day came and we lined up along St Georges Terrace in the downtown area early in the morning. It was cold, much colder than expected. We just wore a running singlet and shorts, so I was freezing. Many of the other runners were better organised and had brought along an old sweater or a plastic bag to wear initially and then discard when the run started. As we were from Singapore, we didn't think to take warm clothing so we stood there close to the front of the group of runners hoping the run would start soon.

I might be a bit biased, but Perth is a beautiful city. It's the capital of Western Australia with 2.1 million people in a state with only 2.6 million people while having a total land area of 2.5 million square kilometres (0.98 million square miles). That's a quarter of the size of Europe. The remainder of the state is sparsely populated.

Aboriginal Australians have lived in the Perth area for at least 38 000 years, as evidenced by archaeological records. The Noongar people occupied the area. Perth is considered the most isolated capital city in the world and one of the windiest along with Wellington, New Zealand. It's typically also rated as one of the most liveable cities in the world. The city centre of Perth is situated adjacent to the beautiful Swan River and that's where we were standing. Twelve kilometres away are the white sandy beaches and clear blue waves of the Indian Ocean.

The marathon route that year took runners around the river to the south past the University of Western Australia, to Nedlands and back through the university, into the city centre and up to Kings Park. Kings Park is one of the world's largest, most beautiful inner-city parks and is home to the spectacular Western Australian Botanic Garden which displays over 3000 species of the State's unique flora. It overlooks the city and Swan River. Two-thirds of the 400-hectare park is protected as bushland and provides a haven for native biological diversity. The race would then weave its way through this beautiful park and back again to the entrance before following a route out through the suburbs to the coast and rolling surf at City Beach.

Maria and I started well. Maria ran a personal best for 10 kilometres, then 20 kilometres, then the half-marathon. The highlight of the run back from the University of West Australia via Matilda Bay was that we passed the iconic Crawley Edge Boatshed and the Eliza bronze sculpture with a pod of dolphins swimming alongside bobbing in and out of the water following us, or so it seemed.

Inside Kings Park there was a long gradual upward section heading north where I added some speed and gained about 100 metres on Maria as a pacemaker would to keep the pressure on both of us to stretch our performance. The race continued like this with both of us running well, me not gaining ground and Maria keeping up her pace. As we ran down the final downhill section into City Beach and turned into the home straight, I looked around and Maria was still only 100 metres behind. At 42.1 kilometres (26.1 miles), we were just 100 metres apart. The finish line loomed up ahead and as I ran closer, I realised that the time was going to be, for the very first time, a PB and a BQ for me and a new PB and BQ for Maria. And so, it was after six years of training, sweating in Singapore, doing intervals, cycling, and running races, I had finally achieved the BQ that I'd been looking for. Maria for the first time lowered her time to three hours and thirty-seven minutes or an average of five minutes eight seconds per kilometre over 42.195 kilometres (26.2 miles).

For that year, we just had the Singapore Marathon left to run. It would be our last in the country and we wanted to make it a good one. Doing well in a race is a great motivator for the next one. It's like a golfer hitting that perfect tee shot or a tennis player hitting a perfect serve. As soon as we got back to Singapore, I checked on what we needed to do to register for the Boston Marathon the following year now that I finally had a qualifying time. The Boston Marathon then had a set registration process that requires people to start the registration process on a set date in September the year prior to the race. Over time the process has improved to allow it to be fairer. At the time, however, it was a first-in process and by the time we registered, given the time difference between

Boston and Singapore and some delays from me, the race had filled. We missed out on getting a place despite our qualifying times. In retrospect this was good as we would be moving back to Australia by then and there would be many things to organise and new jobs to settle into.

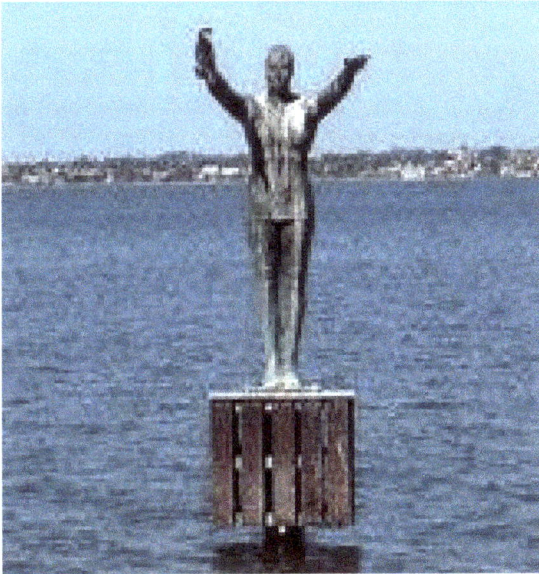

Eliza sculpture — Matilda Bay, Swan River, Perth

The rest of the year went by and Maria moved back to Perth towards the end of the year to take up a new role in an accounting firm. I stayed for a few extra months in Singapore to recruit a replacement and complete a work handover. Maria then flew back for the Singapore Marathon which is held on the first Sunday in December. One of the great highlights of the year in Singapore is Christmas time. The decorations around the city, especially the Christmas lights, along the famous

Orchard Road are spectacular. For over thirty years the 2.2-kilometre (1.4-mile) Orchard Road shopping strip lights up like a magnificent tropical garden at Christmas and is a major attraction for Singaporeans and international visitors alike. It has been ranked third in Lonely Planet's list of 'Top 10 Christmas Markets of the World'. It's not surprising then that the Singapore Marathon starts at the top of Orchard Road before dawn near the Tangs Department store at the corner of Orchard Road and Scotts Road. This allows all the runners to see and run under the Christmas lights all along Orchard Road.

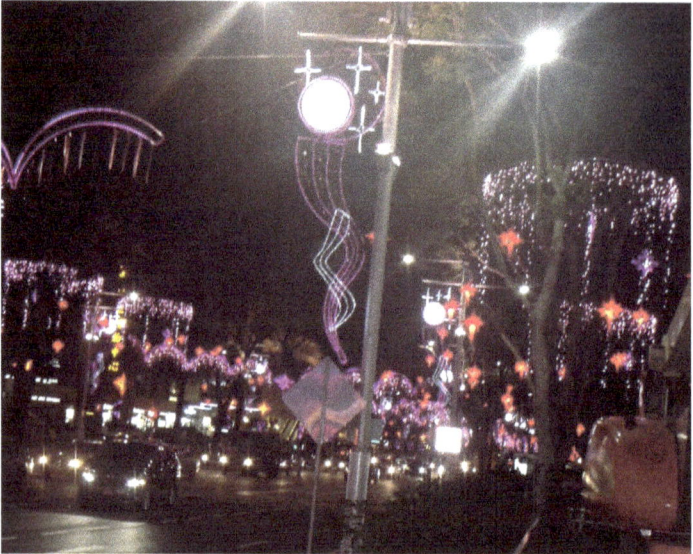

Christmas lights — Singapore

The route of the Singapore Marathon has greatly improved over the years as infrastructure had been upgraded and completed especially in the marina area with the magnificent Marina Bay Sands Hotel and the barrage across the mouth of the Singapore River allowing the race to run further along the coast. In many ways the Singapore Marathon is a guided tour of the wonderful city. It starts at the top end of Orchard Road and goes down to Penang Road past the Dhoby Ghaut subway station and shopping mall, and past Fort Canning out to and through China Town. In just these few kilometres is a mix of colonial, Sumatran, Malay, and Chinese architecture. From there it goes past the famous Fullerton Hotel, the Merlion, out past Little India and then down Arab Street to the East Coast Parkway. Here it passes the East Coast lagoon and then heads back along the coast across the barrage in front of the Marine reservoir and past the Gardens by the Bay finishing in the Padang near City Hall and St Andrews Cathedral.

This time I had trained better. I worked on better nutrition and hydration plans so as I ran the race I did so at a good pace and felt great from start to finish. I was particularly happy with the way I ran the last five kilometres with easy strides, plenty of energy and no cramps. While I finished in a slightly slower time than the recent race in Perth, it was certainly a PB for Singapore and still in the three-hour-thirties time frame. Maria also ran well and like me with a slightly slower time. Overall, in the five years we ran this race, it became better and better organised and had turned into a running festival with 10 km, 21 km, and the marathon races. With that came much larger participation. It was great to see so many people out exercising.

Over the time we spent in Singapore, Maria consistently won almost every race she entered for her age group and she consistently won races for the master's or over- forty group even though she was in her mid-fifties. Often, she would win prizes of running shoes, running clothes or money. For the Singapore marathons she would win a significant cash prize. We joked she could turn professional. She was regularly invited into the elite runners' section to be given a start position at the front of all the competitors. One of the lovely, memorable events we competed in was the Singapore duo 25-kilometre event where a couple, male and female, needed to run 25 kilometres together, totalling 50 kilometres. We won first prize as the fastest couple in Singapore for that event.

*'People take different roads seeking fulfilment
and happiness. Just because they're not on your road
doesn't mean they've gotten lost.'*
— Dalai Lama

Chapter 11

The coldest, most remote place in the world

One day we found ourselves running through soft, uneven sand for 10 kilometres in the searing heat. It was 40 degrees Celsius (104 degrees Fahrenheit). Sweat was running down our faces and even the water in our drink bottles was hot. What were we training for? Was it the Marathon des Sables (MdS) which is French for 'Marathon of the Sands' in the Sahara Desert of Morocco? Were we planning on doing the week long, 251-kilometre (156-mile) ultramarathon, which is approximately the distance of six regular marathons with the longest single stage is 91 kilometres (57 miles) long, a race that has been regarded as the toughest foot race on Earth? Or was it something else?

Back in Perth we settled in quickly and kept the running training going. The year passed quickly. We ran three more races as we prepared for the Antarctic marathon which was approaching the following year. Our run times were good like the year before. During the year, our place on the wait list for the Antarctic marathon was confirmed for the following year. What would it be like running a marathon in Antarctica? Over the New Year period we were in New Zealand visiting our son Elliot and his family, so we went down to the local adventure clothing store which provided clothes, camping equipment and other outdoor equipment for hunting and trekking. We thought the people in the store would be knowledgeable about cold weather as it can get very cold in New Zealand. However, while the staff tried to help, they felt that going to Antarctica and the conditions that we could experience were a long way out of their experience. Nonetheless, they were very helpful and with the guidance from them and others we kitted up for the adventure.

As we lived in a warm climate, we had little knowledge of how to dress effectively for extreme cold weather conditions. After some research and discussing this with people who had lived in very cold climates, we arrived at a few key ideas. Firstly, the purpose of clothing is to keep your core temperature maintained. If your core temperature drops only a few degrees, you can be in serious trouble. Your body will start to shut down. Hypothermia is a fast killer. Secondly, layering clothes is the most effective way to keep warm.

Layer 1 — Polyester or synthetic base layer. This wicks the moisture away from the body. Cotton is no good.

Layer 2 — Wool sweater or material that will absorb moisture from your first layer.

Layer 3 — Light Jacket of either wool or down. Synthetic products and down are lightweight and easy to pack.

Layer 4 — Lightweight Gore-Tex outer jacket and pants. This layer blocks the wind and keep you from getting wet. The Gore-Tex jacket should have a hood as well.

Socks — Layer of thin wool or polyester socks, and then a medium weight wool sock over them. I only used the thin socks during the race.

Gloves — I decided on a thin glove liner with a Gore-Tex over glove. Later my experience skiing in the US confirmed with me that you need to have a liner and a good outer glove.

Headwear — A fleece or wool beanie is best. I also bought a balaclava, a fleece neck covering and a Gore-Tex head covering.

Shoes — I decided on Gore-Tex trail running shoes.

Glasses — There was a very good chance there would be a blizzard (and there was) so we bought ski goggles.

The team from Marathon Tours also provided a clothing list for the times we would spend exposed in the Antarctic during the race and on shore exploring. One comment I noted with particular amusement was the statement 'Jeans are not cold-weather pants'.

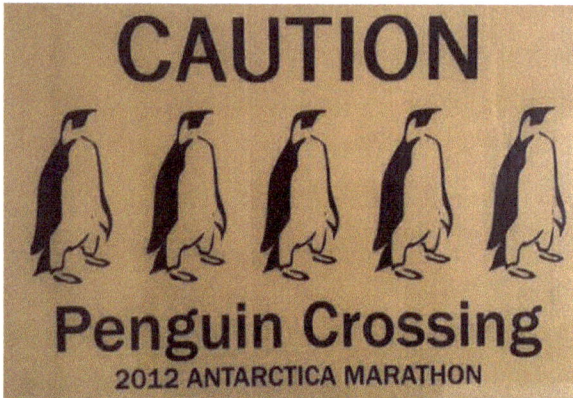

CAUTION

Penguin Crossing
2012 ANTARCTICA MARATHON

As we lived in a hot dry place during summer, we needed to develop a way in which we could train in more challenging conditions, especially to try simulating a run through slush and ice. We finally came up with an idea. On the beach across the road there was about 50 metres of sand between the sand dunes and the sea. At high tide, the water would rise up the beach and cover about fifty per cent of the sand. When the tide ebbed, the sand that was covered in water remained wet and firm to run on. The sand that didn't get wet was soft, powdery, uneven, and challenging to run on, so we decided that we should try to run on this soft, yielding uneven sand to train for Antarctica. It was the only thing we could think of. It's five kilometres from City Beach north to Scarborough Beach so we would run to Scarborough Beach and back on the soft sand totalling 10 kilometres.

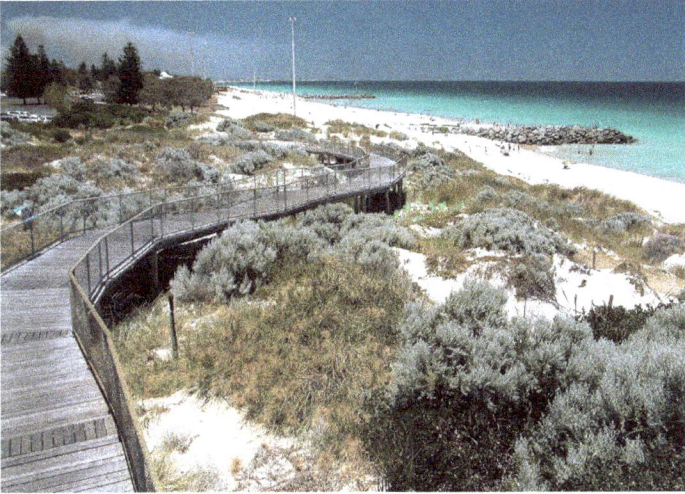

City Beach — Perth

Alternatively, we would run south to Cottesloe Beach and back. We would run at midday on Saturday and Sunday to make the training more challenging. On one run when we reached Scarborough Beach, one person came up to us and asked why we had run so far along the soft sand. Once we explained what we were training to run a marathon in Antarctica. He nodded. 'That makes sense,' he said and walked away shaking his head. I think he thought we were fucking mad too!

The plane flight over was like the travel to Rio De Janeiro several years before as it travelled overnight across the Pacific Ocean from Perth to New Zealand, to Santiago, Chile and then instead of onward to Rio we headed down to Buenos Aires, Argentina. We had never been to Buenos Aires, let alone Argentina, before.

Buenos Aires is both the capital and largest city

169

of Argentina. It's located on the south- eastern coast. 'Buenos Aires' can be translated as 'fair winds'. The city has a multicultural population of around 15.6 million who speak several languages in addition to traditional Spanish. The city's culture has been strongly influenced by European culture so Buenos Aires is sometimes referred to as the 'Paris of South America' with beautiful, graceful architecture which is sometimes characterised as eclectic. It's also the resting place of Eva Perón, Evita, the wife of Argentine President Juan Perón and First Lady of Argentina from 1946 until her death in 1952. We took the time to visit her gravesite and pay our respects as she championed women's suffrage in Argentina, and founded and ran the nation's first large-scale female political party, the Women's Peronist Party.

The group with whom we were going to Antarctica met in a hotel in the city. The organisers and Tom Gilligan introduced themselves at a briefing. Tom was the business owner of Marathon Tours. I recall vividly when Tom was introduced, the speaker commented that why would anyone want to go on board a vessel at sea with someone called Gilligan. This comment referred to the long running US television comedy series called 'Gilligan's Island'. During what was supposed to be a three-hour tour, the charter vessel, the S.S. Minnow, got lost off the coast and all the crew and passengers were shipwrecked on an uncharted tropical island following a typhoon.

The race organisers described what lay ahead for us

over the coming adventure. They also addressed safety and introduced the doctor who would be on the vessel plus the scientist who would provide lectures and discussions on the fauna of the Antarctic especially the marine life like penguins, seals, orcas, and whales. We hoped we would see all of these during the trip. There were significant safety issues to be considered on such a trip and thankfully the organisers and ship's crew seemed to have these covered. For us, sea sickness was a consideration and many people had tablets for this. On Antarctica environmental controls were critical and strictly enforced. Items of clothing especially shoes needed to be cleaned so that no foreign objects were left on the mainland. Nothing was to be left on the mainland including any plastics, bottles, clothes, food, even urine. The critical aim was to keep Antarctica pristine.

It was the first time since the Egyptian marathon that we reunited with our friend from Oman. He was there for the marathon and he too had been captivated by the Seven Continents quest. After the briefing, we and a new friend, Jewel, went off to do a tango lesson which was the traditional dance for couples that originated in this region. So, when in Argentina, tango. Later that evening I asked Jewel how she trained for all the hills of the Antarctic marathon given that she lived in Singapore. She replied that in her training plan she combined runs along the Singapore east coast with stair climbing. In her condominium there was a high-rise apartment block, and she would go to the ground floor stairwell and run up twenty-six floors to the top. So, she was running in the Singapore hot, humid climate up multiple storeys and back to train. Then she would repeat the exercise.

Our next destination was Ushuaia at the bottom of Argentina, the tip of South America. The flight was quick and uneventful. We then had time to look around Ushuaia before we boarded the Akademik Ioffe, a chartered Russian research vessel which was to be our transport for the journey through the Beagle Channel across Drake Passage and along the Antarctic Peninsula at the bottom of the world. With our race confirmation, we were now getting closer to our goal of visiting and running a marathon on the least populated, most isolated, coldest, windiest, and driest continent. In a few days, our Seven Continents quest would be over.

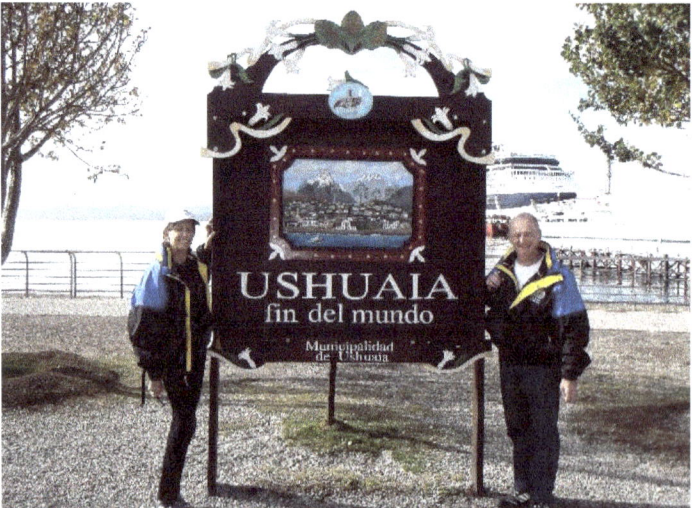

Ushuaia — 'fin del mundo' — end of the world

We arrived in Antarctica after crossing the channel in unusually flat seas. It took two days. We woke in the morning to a very cold, foggy day and could see land off to the south. It looked cold, dark, and forbidding. As we didn't have low-cost internet coverage on the journey, it wasn't surprising to see in the very early morning light, several passengers on deck with their phones trying to pick up a mobile phone signal from the research stations on the shore.

The area we were planning to run is home to four scientific research stations. The land around them is muddy, wet, icy, and windy in summer but suitable for running. The stations are spread out over a 10-kilometre area so it's possible in summer to run between the stations along a track. The environmental regulations were strict with no packaging allowed, all clothes and footwear needed to be inspected and vacuumed and a short six hours' time limit was imposed for the run. Twenty per cent of the 89 participants didn't finish within the time limit but did complete the half-marathon.

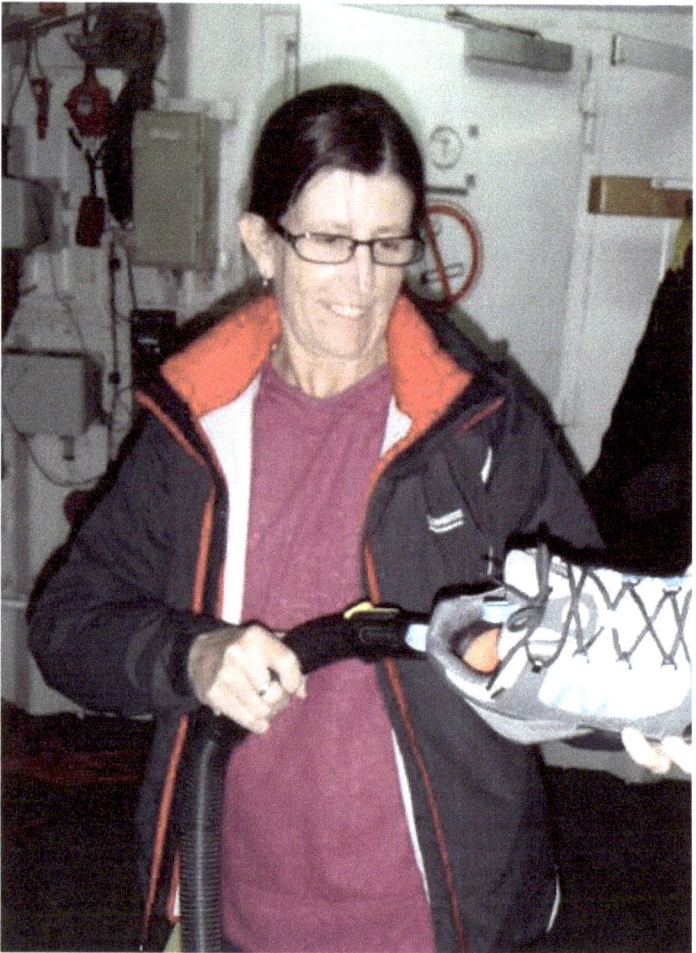

Maria vacuum cleaning her shoes prior to the run in Antarctica

Apart from the weather and terrain the only other consideration was the skuas, *Stercorarius antarcticus* in the ornithological world, which are a group of medium to large predatory seabirds with brown plumage. A skua is typically about 56 cm (22 in) long, and 120 cm (48 in) across the wings so they are a reasonably sized bird and they have the unnerving habit of swooping people and other animals whom they feel are threatening. They reminded me of the masked lapwing plovers which swooped us regularly in my early days when we went running through Limestone Park with my dad. The skuas did do some swooping but were not too threatening or aggressive. One thing I realised well before we went to Antarctica was that there are no polar bears in Antarctica. Polar bears only live in the northern hemisphere in Artic regions.

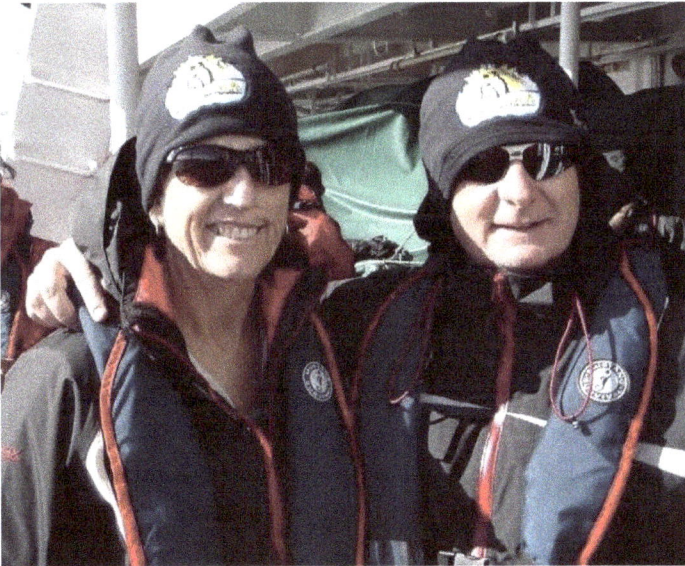

We landed on the shore near the Russian research station and assembled for a briefing. We then started the run and headed off. There was a slight wind, no rain or snow and around -3 degrees Celsius (26 degrees Fahrenheit). This was perfect, much better than expected. It deteriorated quickly however, and within five kilometres the wind picked up, the temperature dropped and it started to blizzard, so when we turned around at the first check point at the five kilometre point, the wind was 60 km/h and the temperature –20 degrees Celsius (–4 degrees Fahrenheit).

As we turned around to retrace the five kilometres back to the starting point, we ran headlong into the blizzard. The terrain was mostly undulating small hills with muddy, icy tracks and lots of slush about, but our footing was good. The main hazards were the blizzard and visibility. Our layered clothing kept us warm and the Gore-Tex shoes provided both warmth and good traction. Not everyone was so lucky. Some lost their footing and were blown over into the mud by the wind gusts. The wind, which came off the glacier, brought even lower temperatures pushing the thermometer down to –30 degrees Celsius (–22 degrees Fahrenheit). This was very cold, but oddly enough, a few years later I experienced colder weather in downtown Montréal, Canada one wintertime.

The route went back to base camp where the Russian and Chilean research stations were located and then headed for five kilometres to the Chinese research station. At this point we had completed ten kilometres into the blizzard since the last turnaround, and it was a welcome relief to turn around and run back with the blizzard on our backs. The slow trudge in the blizzard returned to a run. So back and forth we went until the

42.195 kilometres (26.2 miles) were completed. The finish line was a huge, welcome relief. Maria was first in her age category and was presented with a plaque to commemorate the occasion. We both were presented with Seven Continents finisher medals during a beautiful ceremony back on the ship. It was held on the stern of the vessel overlooking icebergs, penguins, seals, whales, and the beautiful landscape of Antarctica.

The one lesson we very quickly learnt was that your core temperature can drop very, very quickly in such cold, harsh conditions, so we needed to quickly get onto a Zodiac and get back to the ship for some warmth. However, we decided to stay a little while and cheer in some friends. When they arrived, I noticed Maria had her Gore-Tex jacket off and was showing significant signs of hypothermia as she started to shiver uncontrollably, her speech became slurred and she started to suffer from confusion and memory loss to the point she was refusing to put on her Gore-Tex jacket. We quickly sent her back to the ship on a Zodiac together with more runners who huddled to keep her warm. I came back shortly after on the next Zodiac. This hostile environment was no place to stand around passively waiting for runners to finish the race.

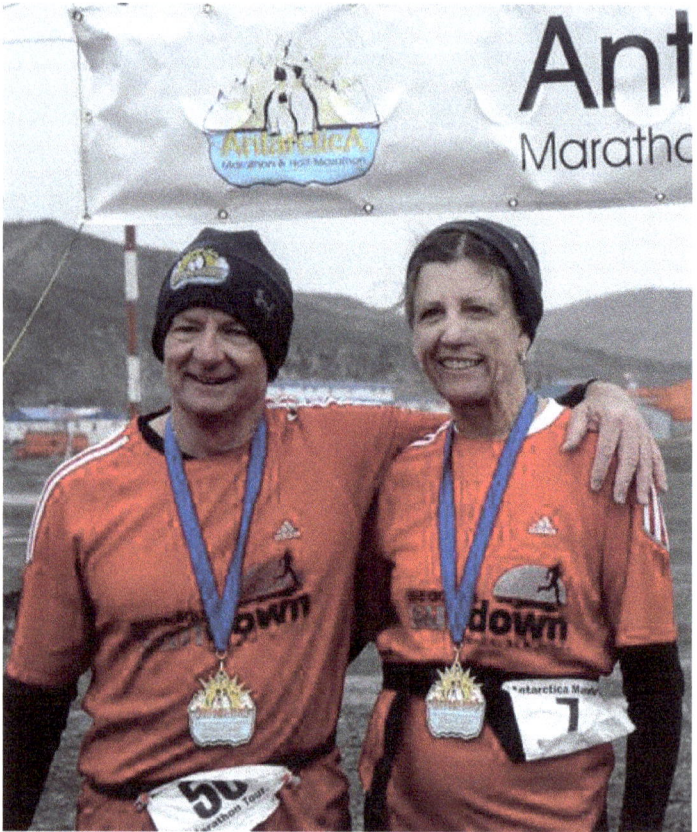

Michael and Maria — after the marathon without jackets

Of course, there were some real characters on the journey with us. One runner wore a chicken outfit for the run to raise money for charity. The same runner took along a surfboard so he could say he surfed in Antarctica. We didn't see any waves and even if we did it would be too cold and dangerous to surf there with the leopard seals prowling in the sea. He did, however, get towed behind a boat around a bay and managed to stand up all the way and end perfectly near the rope ladder at the ship's side. We had another runner who wore his favourite football team's jersey on the run. I'm pretty sure it was an Australian AFL jersey for the Hawthorn Hawks, brown and yellow. His aim was to run every marathon wearing the same jersey.

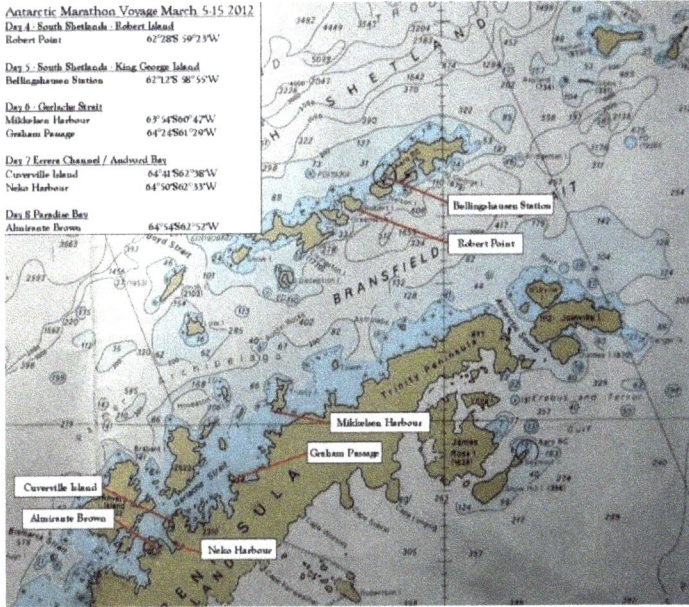

Antarctica Peninsula map

We then spent the remaining six days touring the Antarctic coastline, dropping ashore when possible. We loved the company, scenery, and wildlife including seals, penguins, whales, and orcas. We travelled past Robert Point onto Mikkelsen Harbour, Graham Passage, Cuverville Island and finally to Almirante Brown. One day we passed a pod of orcas chasing some whales. The ship's captain turned the vessel around and cruised after them. It was an amazing spectacle. Several times we got to travel ashore and were dropped off in a Zodiac to view large colonies of chinstrap penguins. At this time of the year you can see the penguins on their nests protecting their chicks from the skuas which love to feed on penguin chicks. The view of the nests offered excellent photo opportunities of the penguins and the rocky surrounds, icebergs, and ice- covered mountains. Access to the area is very restricted and you must not bother the penguins, block their access to the beach or their main paths and you must keep at least five metres or fifteen feet from the penguins.

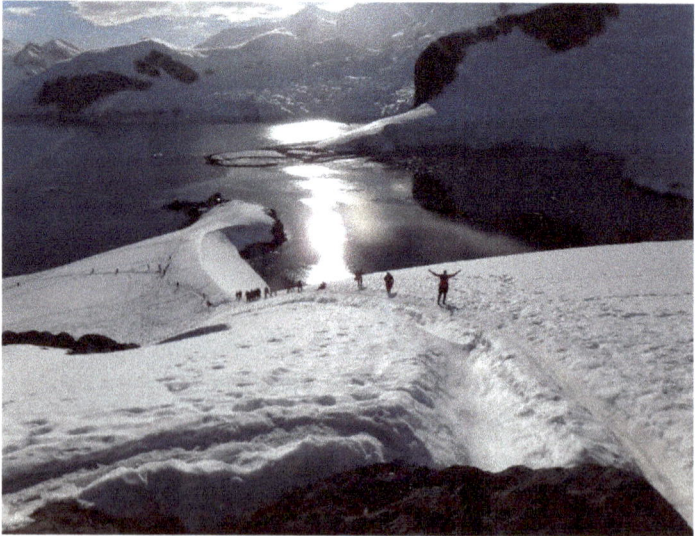

Runners from the Antarctica marathon

It is an amazing region which is teeming with wildlife, seemingly untouched and natural. In one bay where a penguin colony was located several large leopard seals patrolled offshore waiting for penguins to venture out to sea. The penguins would gather on shore waiting for an opportunity to go out to sea and feed. They seemed to know that the leopard seals were present and one or two of the colony would be eaten on the trip out to sea. Eventually one penguin would go into the water and the others would quickly follow believing in 'safety in numbers'. Not all would be able to pass the patrolling leopard seals.

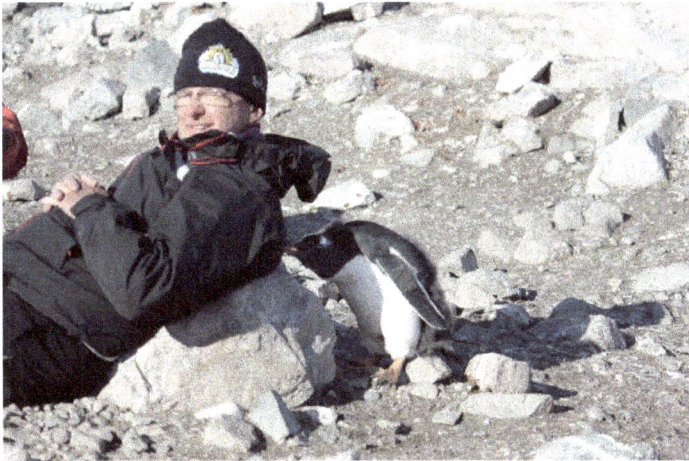

Michael and the inquisitive penguin

The leopard seal is known for its massive reptilian-like head and jaws that allow it to be one of the top predators in Antarctica. It has a silver to dark grey blended coat with a spotted pattern. Its underneath side is pale in colour. Typically, they are 2.4–3.5 metres (7.9–11.5 feet) long and weigh 200 to 600 kilograms (440 to 1,320 lb).

Leopard seals have an enormous mouth relative to their body size and very sharp front teeth.

When we were on the trip the crew emphasised that the Zodiac vessels we would travel around in have a double layer outer skin. There was a rumour that during a previous voyage, a leopard seal came up to the side of a Zodiac loaded with runners and bit the Zodiac, puncturing the side. It then went around to the other side of the vessel and punctured the other side. Thankfully, the Zodiac has a double layer skin and there were other boats around.

By now we had done nineteen marathons on seven continents and had our share of challenges and adventures. We had to run in summer in the soft sand of Perth beaches to train for Antarctica. I collapsed after a particularly gruelling, hot, humid marathon in Singapore. Maria broke her foot halfway through a race in Australia but limped on to finish and spent six months recuperating. We struggled with jetlag, fatigue and disappointment in Rio de Janeiro and ran to near collapse during the hot, final mountain stage of the Great Wall marathon in China. We had also done the challenging Two Oceans Ultramarathon and all these runs were a privilege. We had done some of the coldest, hardest, hottest, and most historic marathons but we were always looking forward to the next challenge.

Chapter 12

Jewel

We met Jewel in Argentina on the way to Antarctica. Jewel is Canadian, a bit shorter than Maria, with long dark hair, athletic, holds numerous academic qualifications and has studied and worked in Nice, Stockholm, New York, Singapore, Moscow, Seoul, and London. Like many people, she downplays what she has accomplished, but behind those dark intelligent eyes you sense the steely determination. Like the lady who I met in Antarctica who decided while watching TV to qualify for, then run the Comrades ultramarathon, Jewel decided to run the gruelling Marathon de Sables (MDS) in the Sahara Desert, Morocco. It is the toughest footrace in the world that I mentioned earlier. One person died and twenty-eight people were hospitalised, airlifted, and in some cases repatriated during the race she ran. If you have ever been troubled by a bit of sand in your shoe imagine running for a week with a one-day double marathon across the rolling sand dunes of the Sahara carrying all your supplies and equipment. This is her story.

If you told me when I was eighteen that at the age of thirty-five, I would be unemployed, single, and living in my parents' basement, I would have killed myself. I don't want to grow up to be a loser! But here I am doing it and I feel like the luckiest loser in the world because living at home for a year will afford me the luxury to train for the biggest adventure of my life yet, one of the toughest footraces in the world, the notorious Marathon des Sables. It's a one-week, six-stage, ultramarathon of 225 km through the Sahara Desert of southern Morocco while carrying a backpack with an entire week's worth of provisions. I hate running. But I have always wanted to see Morocco and I have always wanted to see the desert, so it's a dream come true wrapped in a pretty, near-death experience.

The terrain will consist of baked earth, rocky flats, jagged hills that look and feel more like mountains, and giant mounds of sinking sand dunes that provide the perfect opportunity to get lost. Conditions will be a blazing inferno by day and icebox by night. There will be sandstorms, scorpions, spiders, snakes, sunburn, sleep deprivation, and some degree of starvation to make it extra interesting. On the compulsory list of equipment are things like an aluminium survival sheet, whistle, light, knife, compass, ten safety pins, a signalling mirror, and an antivenom pump. Then there's a mile-long list of suggested items like a pen and paper. What is a spork? What are gaiters? Then there's the list of hazards that reads more like 'Fifty Ways to Die in The Desert'. Some are expected like dehydration, heat exhaustion, heat stroke, cardiac arrest, twisted ankles, falling off a cliff, venomous bites, getting lost, and hallucinating. Others struck me funny like shooting yourself with your own flare gun, kidnapping, getting attacked by camels, and getting run over by a race vehicle. You're in the middle of nowhere! You would think there's plenty of room out there to drive around you, but you could get nailed in the dunes because the vehicles can't see what's on the other side of a mountain of sand. They forgot nuclear war and an asteroid strike.

Last summer I happened to see a documentary on the race and by the time I shut the TV off, I knew I wanted to do it. I also knew I had to quit my teaching job and move back home because I knew training was going to be a full-time job, at least it would be for me. I don't run. I know nothing about it. I don't even own a decent pair of running shoes. My first goal is to survive. My second goal is to finish. Along the way, who knows, I might meet Mr Right in the middle of nowhere and end up married on a potato farm in Slovenia with a dozen kids, or maybe I'll meet a Swiss entrepreneur who wants a pet yak instead of a kid and we'll open up a ski resort for dogs in the Alps. Of course, there won't be any bathrooms or showers out in the desert all week, so we'll have to keep everything at arms' length until we get back into civilisation with a change of underwear and some plumbing. The whole thing stinks of blood and sweat but smells of an epic adventure of a lifetime. How can I not!

Thirty-five Going on Eighty

It's nine o'clock at night and I have my feet up in a recliner in front of the TV, but the TV is off. After a day's worth of goodbye and good luck parties, I finally have a quiet moment to myself in the basement to collect my thoughts with a glass of wine. The wine is here to calm my nerves and hopefully get me to sleep. Tomorrow, I fly out to Morocco.

The last ten months have been bloody awful. I'm supposed to be in the best shape of my life, but part of me feels like I'm going on eighty. Maybe the sofa slugs of the world are onto something. Maybe exercise is for idiots. I thought being in shape was supposed to make you feel like a million bucks, not like a wounded animal that should be put down. I'm exhausted, I ache, I haven't lost a single bloody pound, and my running time hasn't gotten any faster since the day I started. Some people were born to run, like my friends Michael and Maria. After ten months of training, I can see I was born to go slow and suffer. All the training in the world won't make me Usain Bolt. The only thing training has done for me is it's given me the stamina to go slow and suffer for longer periods of time.

My feet have blistered and bled every step of the way. I tried everything on the market, spoke to runners in shoe stores, posted questions on the race website, read a book of 101 solutions, and nothing worked. Band-Aids were a joke. I tried medical gauze, medical tapes, liquid bandages, even electrical tape, and my feet still bled right through my shoes. I tried different shoe brands and different sizes. I tried double socks, dri-fit socks, and toe socks. I tried orthotics. Those just made me blister in new places. I tried foot powders. One burned. One gave me a rash. One itched. I tried corn pads. I tried topical anaesthetics. The shoe 'experts' in running stores had me try different lacing patterns to change the pressure points on my feet. Again, I just got new blisters in different places. One guy told me to lace my shoes tighter to prevent my heels from sliding around so much in the heel box. After a week of that, I got a burning, tingling, bruising sensation on the tops of my feet. I went to my foot doctor and he said it was nerve damage. If I didn't loosen my shoes, the damage would be permanent. So, I had to accept blistering as part of the deal. At the worst of it, all the skin came off both my heels and the balls of my feet with several raw, open wounds in between. My feet looked like two raw steaks. My eyes watered when I walked, but I never quit. I know my feet are going to blister out in the desert, so I thought it best to get used to it now. Besides, it would have taken weeks for my feet to heal and I didn't want to lose the stamina I worked so hard to build up. I refuse to drop out of the race because of blisters because blisters aren't a life-threatening condition, but there were times when I thought I might be the first person to ever die from them.

I also went through several black toes. Some of my toenails bruised from all the banging up against the roof of my shoes. So, they would turn black and then fall off or buckle upward while a new one slowly grew in. Did you know it takes about six months to replace a toenail? And when the nails grew in, I had to let them grow in slightly long, so they didn't become ingrown or need permanently removing. Yes, permanently. Of course, my legs throbbed during the long runs and for hours afterward. I tried taking pain relievers before the runs to soften the pain, but they did nothing. There is no getting around it. The race is going to hurt.

There are plenty of other reasons why training has made me feel like I'm eighty. When you want something bad enough, you will stop at almost nothing to get it, including Depends, those diapers for adults. Before taking on an ultramarathon in the Sahara, I thought I better try a marathon first, so I did New York. The marathon started in Staten Island. Call it nerves, call it I had no idea what I was doing with my fluid intake, but by the time I reached the next borough, Queens, I had to go to the bathroom. So, I pulled off to the side at one of those hideous portable toilet pit stops. It was so disheartening to watch people run by while I stood still in line for a toxic-waste-dump of a bathroom. That cost me a good ten minutes in finish time. I swore never again.

So, I came up with the idea to try Depends. God bless the people who need them for real. I heard runners in the marathon world just go in their shorts, down their legs into their shoes, but I couldn't bring myself to do that. I did see a woman squat between some parked cars, but I have a clean police record. I wouldn't want to soil it with a creepy charge of indecent exposure. I would pick something more glamorous and worthwhile like illegal protesting to stop shark finning. So, I came up with the idea of Depends because it would give me relief without slowing me down for a second.

Step 1: Buy some. Off to the grocery store I went. At 6 am. That's when the store opened and almost no one would be in it. The purchase would be a secret between me and the security guard watching the cameras, and he was probably not someone I cared to impress anyway. So, I dashed into the store full of nerves, but with a plan. I just had to execute it: pick up a large box of cereal, proceed to the Depends isle for a quick grab-and-go, and then head to the check-out stand and place the big box of cereal directly behind the Depends to conceal their view from any midnight-shift customer who might come up behind me. I figured the teenage girl at the check-out would be too half-asleep or too lost in her own world of boys and fashion to notice. I thought it was a flawless plan worthy of a supporting role as Mrs James Bond. I was so wrong.

As soon as I reached the shelf, my eyes grew wide in shock at the expanse of possibilities. So many sizes, shapes, styles, and absorbencies! Words like adjustable, shields, protection with tabs, worry-free odour control, and men's leapt off the shelves. Where the hell are the women's? Damn! I got bogged down in features like I was buying a car instead of a diaper. Focus! Look for the pink! Out of the corner of my eye, I spied a body coming down the aisle. Bloody hell! Quick! Turn to face the baby food! As he got closer, I could see he was not hot, observant, nor conversational, and just after some baby formula. Soon I was alone again. I turned back around, took a few steps down the shelf, spotted some pink on a package, grabbed it, and bolted to the check-out. Fortunately, no one came up behind me. I needed the cereal anyway and the girl was concentrating on the gum she was chewing too much to notice. Thank God she gave me a bag to conceal the deal out to my car. That was stressful. And that was the easy part!

Step 2: Try one. What a struggle! I am horrible at maths, but I excelled at toilet- training. I weaned myself off diapers by the age of two. I had a natural dislike for mess in my pants and I am proud of it. I have spent the last thirty-three years of my life avoiding an accident at all costs, even if it meant rupturing a kidney. So, at the age of thirty-five, it was impossible to drive home, put on a foreign device, and flip a switch in an instant, 'No, it's okay now. You can let loose.' It took two jugs of water and an hour of pacing. When the moment of truth arrived, I went into the bathroom, stood over the tile floor, and somehow managed to let go. So strange, so warm, so soggy, so heavy, so uncomfortable. Now I know why babies cry when they wet their diapers. I wanted to cry too. But mission accomplished. I had to keep the finish line in sight. If Depends was what I had to do to get me through my next marathon, I was willing to do it.

Step 3: Try one out on a twenty-mile run. I wore the biggest shorts in my drawer and the longest t-shirt I could find. I was so self-conscious. I felt like there was a flashing neon sign on my behind telling the whole world 'diaper under here'. During that run I did feel the urge to go, but I just couldn't bring myself to do it. I was in public! What if it leaks? People might see! So, I wore it, but I couldn't use it. When I got home in the shower, I discovered a new problem. Once I got the soap and water running down me, my body quivered. The friction of the diaper combined with the sweat from the run chafed me in the most unspeakable places. Apparently, incontinency products were not designed for long-distance running.

Don't get me wrong. I'm very grateful to the people at Depends for making a product that allows people with genuine incontinency problems to live a normal life. If I lose bladder control down the road when I'm eighty, I will be ever so glad to have them! I just could not bring myself to use them at the age of thirty-five with a perfectly good bladder.

One of the scariest things I experienced during training was chest pain. I was 18 miles into a run when I felt a ton of pressure in my chest like someone was sitting on me while I gasped for air. Then I got a sharp pain in my chest. I panicked. I thought I was having a heart attack, but then I realised the pain was about an inch to the right of my heart so I figured I was going to live, but it scared the life out of me. I didn't want to think about heart attacks for at least another forty years! I stopped running of course and went straight to the doctor. She told me I have exercise-induced asthma and gave me a couple of inhalers to try, but they made me light-headed and nauseous at times. After a few months of hit-and-miss relief, I chose to live with it. I don't care about my time out there. I just want to finish. At least now I know why I hate running. I have been so flaming frustrated because I never cut miles, yet I never seemed to make any progress. Now I know I suck at running because my lungs become too constricted to suck in enough air.

Another reason training made me feel like I'm eighty was the fact that I had medical staff. I thought only old people had more than one doctor and went to appointments all the time. I went to my family doctor for the asthma, antibiotics for foot infections, painkillers, and pre-departure medical tests. I went to a foot doctor to keep an eye on my toenails, the nerve damage, and to try out some orthotics. I went to a chiropractor for all the back pain and the pinched nerve I got from training with the backpack. And I went to my main man Tony, my physiotherapist, for a slight muscle tear and for all the general rigor mortis that set in after long sessions. His steel thumbs hurt like hell, but they tenderised my meat so I could move again.

That's why I had to quit my job. It took me half an hour to get ready for a run. I had to tape my feet, get dressed, and pack my backpack. Then it took a half hour to get to the running path on the Parkway along the Niagara River, Canada. I would run up and down the path between the town of Niagara-on-the-Lake and the flagpole in Queenston. On one side you have the river nestled down below between the clay- coloured, towering cliffs of the Niagara Gorge. On the other side you have lush peach orchards, quaint country fruit stands, vineyards that stretch as far as your eye can see, and boutique wineries. Looked like hell to me. Pain is such a mood-killer. I would do a four-to-six-hour session. Then there was the half-hour ride home. It took me an hour to unpack, shower, and eat because at that point I moved like a black-toed sloth. After that, I was off to an appointment or off to buy more medical supplies. Then it was home to put my feet up in a recliner to try to air-dry my wounds for the next day. I had no time or energy left over for anything or anyone else. For the last ten months, training has consumed my entire life. I just pray it is enough.

Well, I've hit the bottom of my wine glass. I better head off to bed. Instead of moving back home with Mum and Dad, maybe I should have checked into a care home instead for the onsite medical care and sleeping pills. I sure could use one tonight. I hate flying. I'm even more scared to death that I might not finish the race. After all the pain, sweat, blood, money, time, energy, and sacrifice I put in the last ten months, I don't know how I would handle the heartache of coming up short. It would haunt me like unfinished business, but then I don't know if I could ever put myself through all this again. It's now or never. And on that nerve-shattering note, I will now try to get some sleep. I wish we could pre-program dreams for the night. I would order Daniel Craig in his 007 attire with champagne and an eight-course dinner out in a vineyard. I don't want to spend the night running naked through an airport or sinking in quicksand with a herd of angry camels barrelling down upon me. Instead of counting sheep, I will now try to drift off counting rugby players.

Dead but Not Dead

The race was absolutely bloody fucking awful from start to finish as advertised. You can feel yourself slowly rot to death out there as all your major organs slowly shut down under the strain of it all. But I loved it! I've never felt so dead, but so alive at the same time. I felt so sick I spent the last two days of the race pulling into every medical tent begging for an IV, and I hate needles. An intravenous therapy (IV) is therapy that delivers fluids directly into a vein; in this case it would've been a saline fluid. We were allowed one IV for the race so I wanted to cash in and gas up, but I wasn't vomiting or suffering diarrhoea so they refused to give me one. 'No. You will finish,' they said.

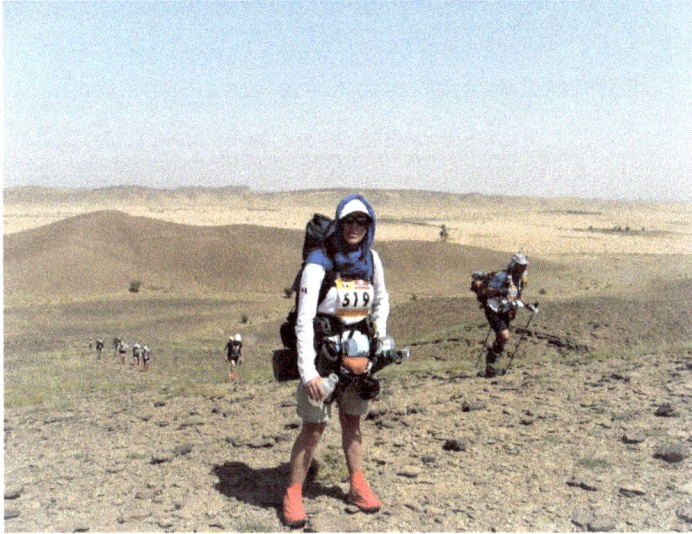

Jewel — Marathon De Sable — Sahara Desert

So, the joy continued. One minute I was hot. The next minute I was freezing, and it was 42°Celsius (108 Fahrenheit). I was starving, but sick of the food I'd brought. It's a desert. You can't bring cheese or chocolate or much else for that matter. So that left astronaut food, that freeze-dried crap, but you can't cook out there so that meant eating rock-hard, uncooked rice or pasta with some flavoured powder on it. Thank God I didn't chip a tooth. Breakfast was a pop-tart and lunch was a power gel and some nuts. By Day 2, just the thought of a power gel made me want to vomit. I had to plug my nose to get them down. By Day 3, I said screw this. I'd rather starve. So, I started giving away my power gels. Why carry them? I knew if I had just one more, I would start vomiting and if I started to vomit, I knew I wouldn't stop, and I'd be out of the race.

Of course, I was exhausted. I was exhausted from the exertion of mile after mile after mile after mile after mile after mile, but I was also exhausted from sleep deprivation. I didn't sleep all week. I was too cold, too hungry, too sick to my stomach, and in too much pain to sleep. So, I got to lie awake all night. Some runners said the scorpions made a clicking noise out there. All I heard was people snore and vomit.

I had four different kinds of pain. Blisters came out in full force, of course. Again, I lost all the skin on my heels and developed gaping holes of raw, bloody flesh on the rest of my feet, but thanks to training I barely noticed. I also developed an absolutely mental throbbing in my legs that started in my feet and progressed all the way up to my thighs as the week went on. It was a pulsating pain that was too deep in the bone to massage. Sitting or lying down gave no relief. Nothing made it stop. I took six pain relievers in one swallow and it still didn't budge so I threw out the rest. Why carry them? Someone said the stuff is hard on the kidneys. By Day 3 I also developed some excruciating pressure that built up in my big toes from all the banging up against the roof of my shoes and one big toe was turning white. Every step felt like someone was pounding me on the big toes with a sledgehammer. The only 'solution' was to cut off the top of my shoes, but then they would fill up with sand in the dunes. Then I would have no skin left anywhere on my feet. Training taught me there's no such thing as a solution, only a trade-off. I had a couple of syringes on me, and I thought I once heard somewhere that if you drill through the nail, it will relieve the pressure. I had just finished the night stage of 80 km, had nothing else to do, and was definitely a bit loopy in the head, but I thought it could be interesting. I got the needle down to a point where I knew I was going to have to shove it down hard to break through and I was worried I was going to stab the needle right into a bone. That was one problem I knew I didn't want. That was the only time I quit out there. As the saying goes, be careful what you wish for. After completing the stage, the following day, I ripped off the medical tape on that white toe and ripped off the toenail with it. I slumped over on the ground and was blinded by a white light. No, it didn't relieve the pressure, but it was exciting to have a new kind of pain to think about. Variety was the spice of life out in race hell. By Day 7, I wanted to die, but there were only 11 km of sand dunes left to the ultimate finish. At that point, I was going to crawl my way there if I had to.

What makes the race so legendary is the race not only wants to destroy you physically but mentally as well. There were plenty of mind games played out there during the week for your entertainment torture. The 'Welcome' tent was empty. 'Nobody cares that you're here. We're not here to help. You're on your own.' The race staff stayed in white tents. They made us stay in black tents. Of course, they absorbed more heat for a human barbecue effect, and they positioned them what seemed like a mile away from the medical tents. Just when you could hardly move, you had to marathon your way to help. The first time I went to 'the butcher shop', I forgot my medical tag. The doctor folded his arms with a smug grin and told me, 'You must go back.' That was a twenty-minute round-trip limp with dizziness and chills. He didn't care. They put mountains at the end of every stage, right when you are on your last breath. They insisted we use the outhouses at camp but put those a mile away from our tents, so you had to marathon your way to the bathroom as well. At one bivouac they put the outhouses on the other side of a sand dune, so we were forced to get sand in our fresh medical dressings. Of course, everyone wanted the bathroom first thing in the morning, but the outhouses were always the first things they took down so if you wanted a bit of privacy you had to get up at 5 am. The cruellest thing they did was disguise a checkpoint like a finish line at the foot of a steep mountain. I was so excited to think I made good time that day, only to discover I was going to have to climb over that mountain for another 10 km while the sun went down. The race staff were lucky that we were too tired to murder them.

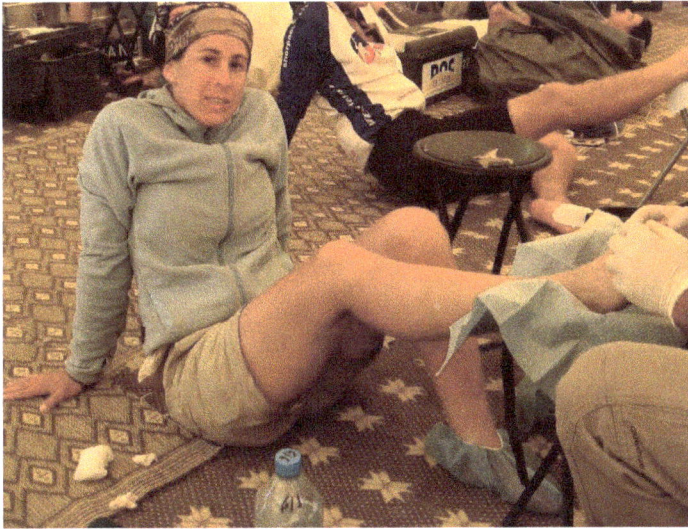

Jewel — in pain while her blisters are cut away and bandaged

But there was good stuff out there too. The world disappeared with all its demands and distractions. That left only the here and now. Nothing else mattered but survival. I was conscious of every moment, every thought, every step, every breath, every heartbeat, and I took none of them for granted. Some say the desert is empty. I was up to my eyeballs in thoughts and possibilities, never-ending space, and freedom. It was quiet and peaceful. You could hear yourself think. You had time and space to connect with yourself, to figure out what you really want out of life when you get back and plan how to get it, time to give thanks for the people and things you have, and time to plan ahead for the future without the aggravating noise of cars, sirens, construction, people, and their bloody phones going off. The desert heightens all your senses and makes life crystal clear, when there's not a sandstorm blowing through.

And then there are all the funny things that go on out there and it's the funny stuff that gets you through. The race is so extreme that the bizarre becomes normal. People cheered when people passed gas out there because that meant that person had body parts that were still functioning. Bravo! My tentmates discussed the solidity of their bowel movements like they were discussing the weather. Solid or liquid? Solid. Really? Good on ya, mate! And I have never seen so many private parts on display going to the bathroom, including my own.

When I signed up for the race, I knew there would be no bathrooms in the middle of the Sahara, but I was too exhausted from training, too stressed out trying to figure out equipment, and too worried about dying to give it much thought. Deep down, I figured the bathroom was something I would sort out when I get there.

It was a five-hour bus ride from the town of Ouarzazate, the final frontier of civilisation, straight into the desert to the start line. Halfway into the journey, all eight buses stopped for a bathroom break. When I stepped off the bus and looked around, I got a huge wake-up call. We stopped in the middle of nowhere. There was the road, a tree, some baked earth, and a steep, rocky barren hill. That was it. Where is the usual roadside umbrella cafe, souvenir stand, and smelly toilets? Nothing. I think it was the race's way of breaking us in for the week. There were 756 of us from all over the world. I got off the bus with a bunch of Canadians, Americans, Aussies, and Kiwis. We all looked at each other like, 'Now what?' Actually, we knew what we had to do. We just didn't want to do it. It figures the Europeans were the first to drop their pants and good on 'em for getting us started. I wasn't quite ready for that so I walked across the road to see what I could find. A culvert! I have never been so excited about going into a ditch. I did my thing and then walked back across the road. When I got to the other side of the buses, the view had drastically changed from an empty desert into a lunar landscape of a different sort. There must have been at least twenty women squatting amongst the men who were in the watering position. Bare backsides everywhere. Then it hit me. I am about to spend an entire week with no pride, no privacy, and no dignity. It was only a matter of time before I would have to drop my pants in front of an audience and there was nothing I could do about it. So, I did the only thing I could do. I took a photo.

Fortunately, the desert broke me in gently. We spent two days in camp at the start line organising ourselves, going through equipment and medical checks, picking up water, and getting to know our tentmates. Nobody wanted used toilet paper blowing through their tent, so the organisers set up two areas of portable toilets. Privacy still prevailed. After the starter's pistol it evaporated quickly.

On Day 1 there was still the odd bush out in the middle

of nowhere, so I used each one trying to empty myself under the scant cover of prickle branches. Bathroom privacy is a terrible thing to waste, especially with so many fit, good-looking men about. On Day 2 bushes were extremely rare and tiny. By Day 3 there was not a single prickle to be found. But at that point I didn't care. I was in so much pain and felt so sick that all I cared about was relief. Not interested? Then look away. I'm going to do what I have to do when I have to do it. When you're in a bad way and doing an ultramarathon, you're not going to hike out of your way. You're going to pull over just a foot or two off the path and drop your pants whenever the fancy strikes you. Sometimes people would ask, 'Ya all right?' Sometimes I would wave 'Hi!' in the middle of it. By Day 4 I didn't care if the race media filmed it. I was in survival mode. So was everybody else. It was the thing to do and the way everyone did it.

Then on Day 5 I experienced co-ed bathroom-going on a whole new level. It was that point in the early morning before the start when the staff had already dissembled the outhouses. There were some small scrub bushes around and you better believe every single one of them had someone squatting behind it. There were already several piles of success left behind from previous squatters. Disgusted? No. Jealous? Yes! I found a vacant bush, dropped my pants, and then tried desperately to take care of some much-wanted business hoping it would somehow make me feel better if I could get things moving.

I happened to glance up from my bush and caught the eye of this handsome guy to the right of me squatting behind another bush trying to do the same thing. He warmly smiled and hollered over, 'Hey!' Time out. Are you kidding me? Is he trying to chat me up? Now??? Think fast! But let us face it. When it comes to flirting, nobody does their best work with their pants down around their ankles trying to make business. I did the best I could. 'Hey!' It didn't end there. Does he know we're not in a pub having a drink? He continued. 'So how ya goin'?' Fortunately, I was still sharp enough to know he didn't mean literally, like he was looking for a play-by-play account of my progress behind my bush. 'I'm hanging in. You?' No matter how miserable you felt, there was an unwritten rule out there, 'thou shall not whine or complain because everyone is hurting, and no one wants to hear it'. 'Good on ya. Yeah, still in it. Just a few more days to go.' He's hot, but he's not helping. What to say? 'Ya, I keep thinking about the finish line and a shower.' 'Ya, the post-mortem party is going to be sweet. Have a good one. I'll see ya later.' Then he got up from his bush, pulled up his shorts, and went back to his tent. I was in no position to go after him. Always my luck.

By the end of the race, I was dropping my pants all over the place and I would have sold tickets. I was in so much pain and felt so sick that I didn't care who saw me. Funny enough, as soon as we got back into civilisation and the bus dropped us off on a sidewalk in the middle of town, I remember feeling I have to go. So, without hesitation I started to unbutton my shorts on the sidewalk. Then a bus went by and it dawned on me. We're back. I have to look for a bathroom now, or at least something with a door. I never thought of civilisation as so bloody inconvenient.

On a more serious note, twenty-eight people were airlifted for life-threatening dehydration, heat stroke, venomous bites, and heart trauma. One man died. He was an amazing runner, in the top fifty for the race. He went full out during the 80-kilometre stage and then took some sleeping pills to settle down that night for some recovery. He never woke up the following morning. His death made us all question why we were there. After all, no one held a gun to our head. We were there because there's something in us that makes us need a challenge like we need food, water, and shelter. It's the thrill of the buzz and the satisfaction of achieving a goal. It's also a bit selfish, so these things need to be about risk management. We all have family and friends who want us home alive and well and in one piece. We all threw out our sleeping pills.

On my last night out in the desert, I wasn't sure if I was going to make it. The last full day out in the desert, Day 6, is always a full marathon. It took me eleven hours to complete the stage because I stopped in every medical tent. Aside from the excruciating pain in my legs, I felt so sick and achy, I couldn't concentrate, was a bit confused, had a hard time putting thoughts together, and I was getting light-headed like I might pass out. They did tests in every tent and kept saying, 'You will finish.' Ya, if I don't wander into Algeria.

I did finish the stage under a night sky. When I got to my tent, I was too exhausted to eat. All I could do was flop down between my tentmates. I tried to go to sleep, but my heart rate wouldn't settle for hours. My heart pounded in my chest like a revved-up engine that wouldn't idle even though I was lying still. I felt like I was teetering on the brink of cardiac arrest, that it was going to stop all together out of sheer exhaustion. That fear only added more stress to an already struggling organ. I kept telling myself I had to stay calm if I was going to make it.

As luck would have it, I had the most handsome tent in the race. Aside from me, there was a married couple, and then six other guys at various levels of commitment. It just so happened that I spent my last night out in the desert sandwiched between the two most handsome guys in the entire race. One looked like an Armani model from the UK and the other looked like Daniel Craig's brother from New Zealand. If I was going to go, I was going to go most happy. Normally I would have found all sorts of yummy thoughts to fill my head, but my heart was pounding up against my sternum. So, I spent my last night out in the desert lying awake in my sleeping bag, shivering, scared, starving, throbbing in pain, praying to God, and fantasising about bread. Sorry, guys. No offense. The desert does strange things to people.

Thank you, God. I survived the night and finished

the race the following day. Some people cried when they crossed the finish line. People cried out there all week for different reasons, including the men. When you're so far gone, your body does all sorts of strange things you don't understand. You feel things you have never felt before because you've never pushed yourself to such an extreme. That was probably the scariest bit about the whole race. You know something is wrong with you and you don't know what your body is going to do next. Are you going to throw up? Are you going to pass out? Are you about to mess your pants? Are you going into cardiac arrest? Should you fire up your flare gun?

I cried once out there, and I am not a crier. From the moment I signed up for the race, I feared being alone out in the desert for the night stage. The sun was going down and my heart was sinking with it. As I entered the sand dunes, there just so happened to be a couple French runners nearby so I slipped into French mode. Lucky for me, I lost my balance and toppled over onto the sunglasses that were still in my hand. My only pair. Of course, they broke. Ah, merde! The French perked up. They came to see if I was okay and they hated to see I was alone, so they adopted me for the night. Viens avec nous! An answered prayer. I lived in France briefly, so we chatted away like old friends, but they went above and beyond the kindness of strangers. They ignored the race and let me set the pace, kept asking if I wanted them to slow down. C'est d'accord? We laughed and chatted and sang under the stars. I got them to belt out 'The Marseillaise' at the top of their lungs. That's the beauty of being out in the desert. What got me in the end was that they offered me food, food that they suffered carrying, food that could cost them the race. I couldn't. I thanked them and said I was fine. When we entered the checkpoint, Eurosport television was there and stuck a camera in our faces. I stood next to our fearless leader who explained how we met. Then they asked me to say a few words in English. I lost it. I don't know if it was exhaustion, relief, or the compassion these people showed for me. They were humanity at its best. I just started crying on his shoulder for all the world to see, one of my most embarrassing moments captured for all of posterity. They even put it in the official race video for that year so all the other runners could see, including my tentmates, including the guy at the bathroom bush. How lovely. Maybe I shouldn't be embarrassed. I don't know. I'm still trying to process it. I might never understand it. Thank God the other French guy started crying too! That's the beauty of the race.

When I crossed the finish line, I was numb. I was too tired and probably too dehydrated for tears of joy. I was too tired to feel anything. It seemed so anticlimactic. One foot over the finish line and the whole ten-month epic journey came to an end, just like that. No bells or whistles or fireworks. They put a medal around our neck and a bag of food in our hand. In it was a giant hunk of bread! If I felt anything, it was relief. I've had enough, thank you.

Where's the shower? I had to get wheelchair service for the flights home.

When I got back from Morocco, it took me a month to recover. I don't remember the first week because I was strung out on painkillers. All I did was drift in and out of consciousness in between pills while sprawled out like roadkill in a recliner. After a month, the pain finally subsided but the slightest bit of physical exertion exhausted me. I didn't care or complain. I was just thankful to be alive and thankful I didn't need surgery or have anything permanently removed. I got the skin back on my feet and eventually all my toenails too. Eight out of ten went black out there. Overall, it truly was an experience of a lifetime. Now it was time to get on with life.

Now what?

Running is a dark, evil vortex. The danger of showing up at events like these is meeting people. These people are cool. They do things. They go places. They know stuff. They plant evil seeds in your head about signing up for another God-awful, borderline stupid, sick event that is going to cost a mint of money and a world of hurt. The problem is, I am a sucker for 'interesting'. While out in the Sahara, on Day 2 of the race, I overheard some other runners talking about a marathon in Antarctica. I've always wanted to see Antarctica and, as much as I hate running, doing a marathon there seemed like the best up-close and personal way to see it. Marathon Tours billed it as 'The Last Marathon' so I thought it was the perfect way to hang up the marathon shoes for good. When my name cleared the waitlist two years later, I found myself living in Singapore so I had to train for Antarctica in the heat and steam of the equator, but I had already trained for the Sahara in the deep-freeze blizzards of winter in Canada. Note to all single men out there: I swear running is the only dysfunctional part of my life. As long as I suffered, I knew I would be fine.

Everything about Antarctica was more than I could ever imagine. Me, this wounded animal in running shoes who hasn't got a clue, got sponsored by my school, Ngee Ann Secondary School, in Singapore to do the race. I thought only professional runners got sponsored, runners who stood a chance at winning. I tried to explain to my principal, Mr Adrian Lim who was an exceptional leader, that the only way I will win is if everyone else gets lost or dies. I told him I don't know if I will even finish. He didn't care. The school rented out an entire sports facility to hold a one-day running event starring me that was covered by The Straits Times newspaper to raise $25 000 for needy students. Never in a million years did I think my running could ever help someone else. On top of that, I actually won my age category for the marathon in Antarctica. There were only seven of us! But somewhere in a box in my parents' basement is a plaque that says I came in first for running.

It was at that race that I met Michael and Maria. Technically, we met at the briefing in Buenos Aires,

Argentina, but it was through Antarctica that we got to know one another. I remember having breakfast with them on board the ship one morning and Michael asked me if I knew about The Seven Continents Club. Huh? Michael said I should think about doing it because I'm doing the toughest leg of it now. I've already got North America (New York) and Africa (Morocco) in the bag. Damn! Damn! Damn! Damn! Damn! Antarctica was supposed to be my last. It's called the last. I told all my friends and family it would be the last. Like I told you before, the danger of showing up at these things is meeting people. Michael made The Seven Continents Club sound so interesting and so doable at this point. I was already living in Singapore so I could knock off Asia when I get back. How can I say no? Damn the people at breakfast! (Thank you for changing my life, Michael!) Others were chiming in with events to do, things that might suck me into more suffering. That's when I said, 'Everyone shut up about doing stuff!'

So, I went on to run Singapore's Sundown Marathon that Michael already told you about. Of course, for me, it turned into the sunrise marathon with my finish time. We had a vicious thunderstorm during it. At the 30 km mark, the route passed by my bedroom window. I cannot tell you how tempting it was to go home with lightning striking all around and rain pelting me head to toe, but now I had a finish line beyond the finish line to keep me going.

Then it was down to Sydney to knock off Australia. It was so nice to do another event with Michael and Maria and some other Antarctica friends. Maria beat me by an hour with a broken foot! The beginning of the race was beautiful, running over the 'coat hanger' bridge and through a park. I do, however, remember Sydney for its switchbacks. There were several rows of them out in a non-descript part of town. It was so mental seeing runners just 50 metres over who were actually three kilometres ahead of me. But I love you all the same, Sydney. It's one of the most iconic finish lines in the world at the Opera House.

Next, I did Rome to check off the box for Europe. That one starts and finishes at the Colosseum. Like any big city marathon, it had its stunning bits and its monotonous bits. I packed a coin in my belt to throw in the Trevi Fountain along the way, but from the running route I would've had to toss it over the heads of hundreds of people and I didn't want to risk taking someone's eye out. It was also right about there that the cobblestones were doing my head in, not to mention my legs. Ma, molte grazie Roma!

I finished the seven continents in Rio de Janeiro, Brazil. Michael has already given it a thorough go over so I will only add that for me, personally, it was the most beautiful marathon in the world, probably because that one really was my last! I will say, if you're only going to do one marathon in your life (good luck with doing just one), Rio is a good one to do because it's a straight 42 km up the coast along some of the most iconic beaches in the world. Tudo bem!

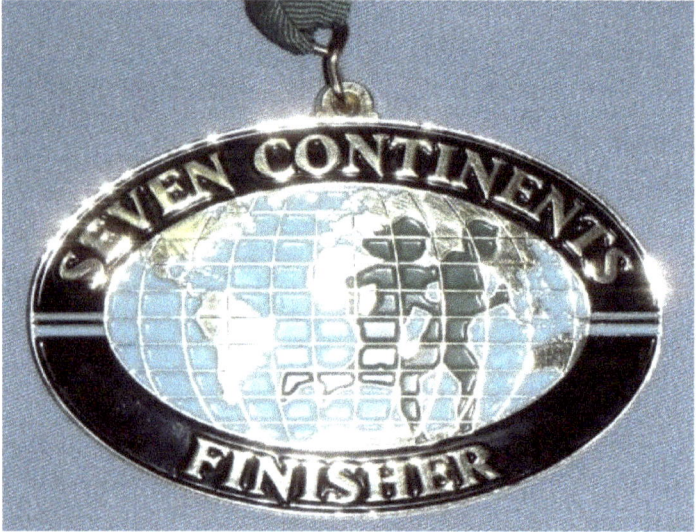

Seven continents marathon medal

When I crossed the finish line, I did have a bit of water in my eyes. Never in a million years did I think I would run my way around the world, so to speak. Never in a million years did I think I would ever belong to such an exclusive running club. If you take that first step, you'll be amazed at where it will take you.

'So, go ahead. Change your life.' — Jewel

Chapter 13

You are always on my mind

'Always on My Mind' is a love song written by Wayne Carson, Johnny Christopher, and Mark James. It was first recorded by BJ Thomas in 1970, first released by Gwen McCrae in 1972 and also released by Brenda Lee, Elvis Presley and John Wesley Ryles. Willie Nelson released his version in 1982. I love Willie Nelson's version. That version held a special place and time in my life when I was first married, however, the words accurately reflect some other thoughts I had at this time. Once you achieve one goal another one appears. Now it was the Boston Marathon that was 'always on my mind'.

During the previous year Maria suffered a stress fracture in her foot. She didn't know it at the time, but she entered the Perth Marathon and aggravated the injury during the race. She did complete the race but then had to seek medical help. She never thought of withdrawing from the race, but she ended up spending several months recovering on crutches.

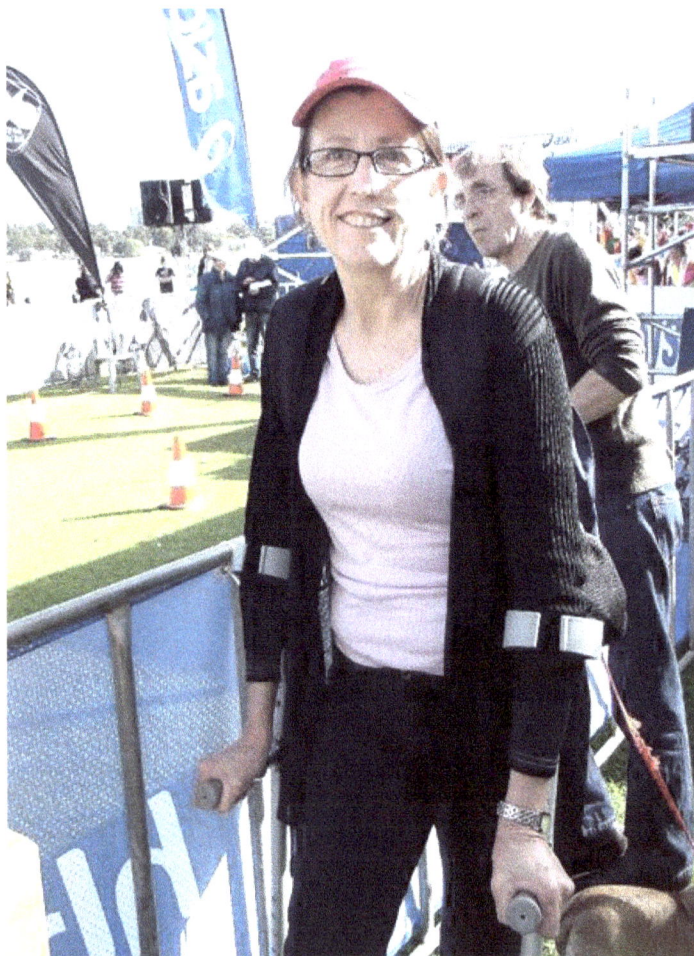

Maria — on crutches in Perth

After the Antarctic Marathon we again completed several marathons that year. It was a short 10-kilometre (6-mile) race in which Maria tripped and ended up with a fracture in her other foot. Again, she was back on crutches. We were concerned that there was some underlying issue as she had a fracture in each foot inside a year. We questioned low bone density or over training, but nothing was conclusive. Her medical specialist advised against running ever again.

Later that year, our friend from Qatar and Jewel came over to Sydney for the Sydney Marathon together with two other friends that we met in Antarctica. One was from New York, USA and the third was an Australian from Victoria. For all of them it was to be the Australian leg of their Seven Continents challenge. For our friend from Oman it would be his final marathon for the Seven Continents. Maria was still recovering at the time and had been off crutches for a month, but she hadn't done any training. She was still signed up for the race and waiting for race day to see how she felt. She figured she had eight years of good quality marathon training and racing behind her and felt that if the foot felt reasonably good, she would run. She was not expecting a great time but felt confident. I think she simply didn't want to miss out on the opportunity to do a marathon in Sydney which required significant effort and travel.

Race day arrived and Maria put on her running gear. She was ready for the race. We trotted over the Sydney Harbour Bridge to the starting line in North Sydney at Bradfield Park, Milsons Point which was immediately adjacent to the Harbour Bridge off Fitzroy Street. A large crowd of participants had gathered as it was part of the Sydney Running Festival plus it was an opportunity to run around Sydney and see all the historical, famous, and spectacular landmarks like Centennial Park, Royal Botanic Gardens, The Rocks, Circular Quay and the many stunning views of Sydney Harbour. The start point was also a great photo opportunity with Sydney Harbour and the Sydney Opera house in the background which would host the finish line.

The race went well. Our friend finished his Seven Continents Challenge, Maria finished in an outstanding time considering her lack of training and so did the other friends. I hit a long-term target of averaging exactly five minutes per kilometre over the 42.2 kilometres. I had a new PB and BQ.

In September that year I received an unexpected early morning phone call from a colleague in Melbourne. He advised me that a sister company wanted to know if I was interested in applying for a role in the US, based in Denver, Colorado. I had visited there many times over the years on company business. Maria had also been there many years before.

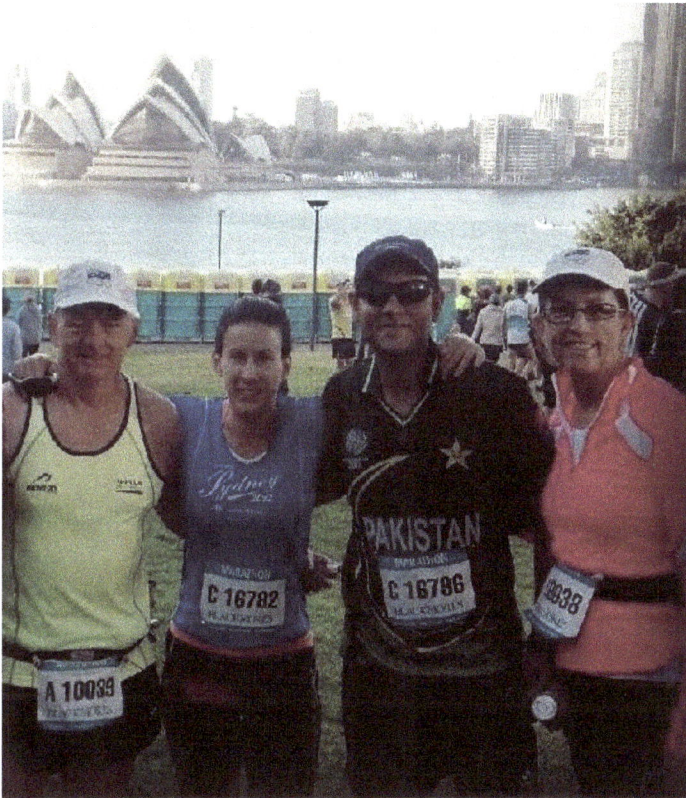

Michael, Jewel, a friend, and Maria in Sydney prior to the race.

I spoke with Maria about the move and she thought it would be a great place to live and an interesting thing to do if not a great life experience, so I applied for the role and was successful. Consequently, shortly after the Sydney Marathon, I found myself in Denver starting a new role and at the beginning of a transition process that would see me phase out of my old role and move into the new one. We had moved many times in the past so we knew the process and realised that it would take time

217

to find a new place to live, buy a car and settle in but we also knew that it was manageable. Saying goodbye again to family was difficult, but I knew it would only be a three-year assignment and a great opportunity to live in the USA which is something we had always wanted to do. It would also offer the opportunity for members of the family to visit and tour around the US.

One of the first things we did after moving to Denver, settling into work, and finding a townhouse to live in was to look for a running club. In our research we discovered three things. The main road running club was the Rocky Mountain Road Runners which was based in Denver near where we lived. We found that there are a lot of marathons run in the US plus it's quick and inexpensive to travel.

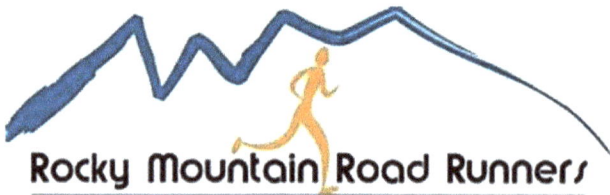

Rocky Mountain Road Runners

We did join the Rocky Mountain Road Runners (RMRR) who were a wonderful, welcoming group. They organised monthly runs in various locations, ran a weekly interval training session when the weather was favourable and organised a marathon training program involving several weeks of organised long-distance endurance runs. Although the RMRR had an interval training session it wasn't convenient for us. I found the Phidippides Track Club which we joined a year later in Denver.

Shortly after we settled into Denver, the New Year arrived, and I received a message from our friend in Oman. He was planning to do the Los Angeles Marathon which was to be run on St Patrick's Day, the 17th of March and he wanted to know if we could join him. This gave us less that ten weeks to prepare. It was winter when I received the message. There was a foot of fresh snow on the ground. I remember we got into the car one evening to find the nearest park, which was Washington Park. When we arrived, it was completely covered in snow so deep that we could not locate the path to run on. So, we had to abandon that training run. In a few days, the snow was gone, and we experienced some of Denver's beautiful winter days with green grass and clear blue sky. It was cold, but running was now back on the agenda. We quickly established several running routes including past the Denver Country Club and around Washington Park, around Cheesman Park near the Denver Botanic Gardens and around City Park near the Denver Zoo. As we lived in Cherry Creek, we also ran along the creek on the pathway either towards the city centre or in the opposite direction towards the Cherry Creek reservoir. A friend also recommended that we purchase some Yaktrax Walk Traction Cleats for the bottom of our shoes to help prevent slipping on ice when we were running or walking. These proved to be invaluable.

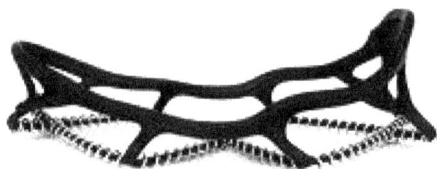

Traction Cleat

Later in March we met our friend in Los Angeles at the Biltmore Hotel which is famous for being used as the venue for the Oscars from 1930 to 1943. The hotel also had been frequently used as a location for film scenes in various movies including the first *Beverly Hills Cop* movie, *Pretty in Pink*, *Rocky III*, *The Sting*, *Ghostbusters*, *Alien Nation*, *The Fabulous Baker Boys*, *Cruel Intentions*, *Bugsy*, *The Fan* and *Bachelor Party*. The famous film director Alfred Hitchcock used the Biltmore's eleven-storey high back staircase for the vertigo sequences in his 1958 movie of the same name. It was good catching up with our friend again.

The marathon started at the Dodger Baseball Stadium in Los Angeles. We were fortunate as the stadium was open for the runners to see. It's magnificent. The route left the stadium carpark went down through Chinatown, past Central Los Angeles, Hollywood, West Hollywood, Beverley Hills, Westwood and ended at Santa Monica near the pier and beach. As it was St Patrick's Day the Irish were out in force. At some locations, they were offering free beer to the runners! It was a wonderful run and a lot of the locals who saw us after the run gave us a high-five and 'Good job!' welcome to California. Our times were slower than our new normal but still good after training through winter. We were again encouraged with the running and booked a range of races which allowed us to periodically travel to various locations and race. The flights were inexpensive and convenient so we could fly out on a Friday night and come back Sunday.

Shortly after the LA Marathon a friend of ours from the Antarctic marathon contacted us and to say he would be coming to Denver in August to run Pikes Peak which is billed as America's Ultimate Challenge and the second most challenging marathon in the world. We invited him to stay with us and then set about trying to enter the race ourselves.

The Pikes Peak Ascent and Marathon is a trail running competition that begins at the base of Pikes Peak, in Manitou Springs, Colorado, and involves over 2382 metres (7815 feet) of relentless climbing to the top of the 4302 metre (14 115 foot) peak.

Manitou Springs is just south of Denver and Pikes Peak is a mountain in the Rocky Mountains. Since 1956, the event has taken place in late summer. There's an Ascent of 21.1 kilometres (13.3 miles) which takes place on the Saturday and the marathon takes place on the Sunday. The marathon is a run up the mountain and back. Some people do the Ascent on the Saturday and the Marathon on the Sunday.

Because of the nature of the run (dirt trails, rock, and other natural obstacles) and the high altitude, the race is much more difficult than standard 42.2-kilometre (26.2-mile) marathons. The average grade of the slope is eleven per cent with some sections much steeper and some flatter. The initial 5 kilometres (3 miles) are very steep. The central 11 kilometres (7 miles) is rolling rocky terrain and the top 4.8 kilometres (3 miles) is above the tree line and require some rock scrambling to reach the summit. Oxygen levels decline as altitude increases and the steep running make the race an extreme event. The weather in August is also variable. In some races it's hot and dry. During others there has been snow at the peak.

At that time, the Pikes Peak Marathon had a qualifying process for which the runners needed to have completed a registered marathon in under four hours. This may have changed since we ran it, but it was the required standard at the time we applied. I assumed that as the race was so demanding the race directors only wanted reasonably fit people to race. I heard that some people had died from the exertion on the run. Sadly, this was not unusual as this had occurred twice before in races, we had competed in. One was a 42-year-old man who died during a triathlon in which I was competing in Singapore. He had a cardiac arrest during the swim leg and while the officials were very quick to commence aid he sadly died. Another had occurred in the SAFRA half-marathon in Singapore where a runner collapsed after the race.

Even though we had a qualifying marathon time the

race numbers had been filled. The race attracts hundreds of runners for both the ascent and for the marathon. The USDA Forest Service limits the number of runners to 1800 for the ascent and 800 for the marathon, and the race registration typically fills in one or two days. The organisers, however, offered us an alternative entry mechanism which was that we needed to participate in the Triple Crown Race Program which involved three races and one was the Pikes Peak Ascent. The first was The Garden of the Gods Ten Mile race. This is a spectacular but physically demanding course, through the incredible Garden of the Gods Park which lies between Manitou Springs and Colorado Springs, Colorado. The second was the 12-kilometre Summer Roundup Trail Run. We completed the two races and then had entry into Pikes Peak marathon for August which was held in the front-range area near Manitou Springs.

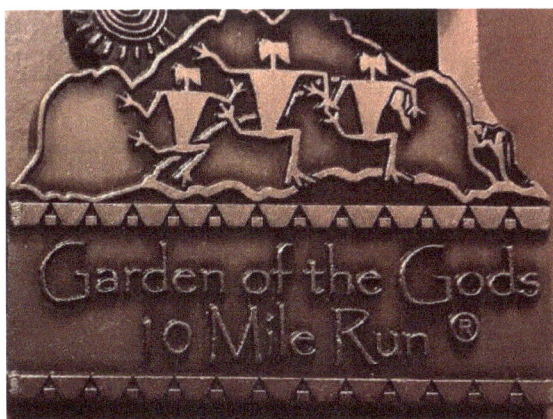

My 'Garden of the Gods' medal

After the LA marathon we registered for the Seattle Rock and Roll Marathon in June, the Chicago Half-Marathon in July, the Montréal Marathon in September, and the Denver Marathon in October. Together with the LA Marathon and Pikes Peak this would make five marathons for the year and one formal half-marathon in Chicago. It was also three marathons in three months. The aim was to also get some BQ results that we could use the following year to run the Boston Marathon. BQ results were valid for two years.

Now that we were in the US, running the Boston marathon was always on my mind.

Chapter 14

Pikes Peak — America's ultimate challenge

We were sitting in our car by the South Platte River on the north side of Denver on a Saturday afternoon and were bamboozled, if not lost. Our first Rocky Mountain Road Runners race was scheduled for the next day and since we were new to Denver, we went out to make sure we could locate the starting point for the run. Being from Australia, we were not used to the grid pattern of the road system where a road could run for very long distances. We did not own a GPS at the time and smartphones were still not the norm. I owned a Blackberry phone, not a smartphone, and it didn't have a GPS nor applications that I could work easily. The avenue system of naming roads was great when you got used to it but today, we were confused as some of the roads were so long that they never seemed to end.

Take for example Coalfax Avenue, a main street that

runs east–west through the Denver metropolitan area. In 2006, the first Colorado Colfax Marathon was held, traversing the length of Colfax Avenue for 42.2 kilometres (26.2 miles). The legend is that one magazine called it the 'the longest street in America'. It took a while to realise the reason that we were lost was that we were looking for an address on S Santa Fe Drive where the Platte River Bar and Grill was in Littleton in the south. But we were many kilometres away at the wrong end of the road and for some reason the house number we were looking at was the same. After some thought we realised our error and drove across town to Littleton, found the correct address and we did make our first Rocky Mountain Road Runners' race the following day. It was a beautiful run alongside the South Platte River. Over the coming years we would regularly run half-marathons, train, and ride our bikes along the river. Even in winter with the snow and ice it was a beautiful place.

The next destination was Seattle. Seattle is a seaport city on the northwest coast of the United States and is the largest city in both the state of Washington and the Pacific Northwest region of North America. It's a lovely city. The St Jude Rock 'n' Roll marathon started and finished in a park near the city centre where the Space Needle is located and is adjacent to the Seattle Monorail Centre Station. The race was amazing, well supported, well organised, and ran along a beautiful course. The lakes and water ways in Seattle are magnificent making it a picturesque course.

We both ran well in great times. Maria finished second in her age group and was pleased with her run.

There was one very memorable part of the race for me. As we ran through Woodland Park and then along Green Lake, the city had put up on the side of the road an American flag for every service person from the local area who had died in the line of duty. The flags lined the entire side of the road adjacent to the lake for miles. It was a very moving memorial to the sacrifices these people had made for their country. In Perth we have a similar memorial in Kings Park. Alongside the roads that traverse the park are ghost gum trees. These are tall eucalyptus trees with a distinctive white trunk and at the foot of each tree is a memorial plaque for a local military person who died for their country. Appropriately, most of the memorial plaques and the trees were placed there by a relative who was typically the mother. In some cases, there are memorial plaques for multiple service people from the same family which is very sad.

We both really enjoyed visiting the city and doing a few tours. We even found a wonderful restaurant down on the waterfront called Elliott's Oyster House. It has the same name as our son so we figured it must be great and it was with good service and seafood.

After Seattle we travelled a few months later to Chicago to run the half-marathon. While we normally run a half-marathon or more in training every weekend, we decided it was a good excuse to travel to Chicago and visit the city in summer. I had been to Chicago a few times before but always on business and in winter when it was very cold with the wind was blowing off Lake Michigan. No wonder Chicago is called the 'Windy City'. Chicago in summer, however, is amazing and we had a great time and even ended up in a great jazz club one evening. While Chicago was not the birthplace of jazz it was one of the early places where jazz took off with musicians like Louis Armstrong and Jelly Roll Morton. We particularly loved the foreshore area around Millennium Park, Grant Park and the Buckingham Fountain which is one of the largest fountains in the world. The fountain was donated by Kate Buckingham in memory of her brother Clarence. In 1925 Kate also gave Clarence's famous art collection to the museum along with an endowment to maintain and expand the collection which has grown from 2500 works to more than 16 000. We took the time to see and admire that famous art.

The next race was Pikes Peak Marathon in August. We didn't realise it at the time, but the race is considered, among endurance runners in the US, an event that they aspire to do but many don't because it's too daunting. Running up 2382 metres (7815 feet) from the start, climbing over 21.2 kilometres (13 miles) in an environment with depleting oxygen was just too much for some. For others, like us, it was a must-do event. The top is just over 4302 metres (14 115) feet. For Australians Mt Kosciuszko is 2228 metres, or for Europeans Mount Mont Blanc is 4810 metres.

Just weeks before the event at Manitou Springs, the race starting point suffered a significant rain event which resulted in a mud slide into the town centre, so when we arrived, we could still see the impact areas from the mud slide. Despite this natural disaster, however, the ever-resilient town's folk and event organisers had reorganised things and the race ran extremely well. You could tell that it wouldn't stop them from putting on America's second oldest marathon. I still felt for the business owners though who had mud in their premises and suffered from blocked access areas.

Our friend arrived from San Francisco on the Friday before race weekend. He was an Australian and a very accomplished marathon runner. While being an amateur he could still run a two-hour forty-minute marathon. We realised after he arrived that he has registered for the Ascent on the Saturday only and not the marathon on the Sunday. We were running the marathon. So, Saturday morning we travelled together down to Manitou Springs so he could run his race. After doing some research we found that the course record holder was Matt Carpenter whose record was two hours one minute for the Ascent and three hours 19 minutes for the marathon. These were very impressive times. Our friend's race went well but as he was living at sea level, he found the altitude extremely tough. He was completely exhausted and out of breath at the top of the mountain when he finished.

The next day it was Maria's and my turn. It was nice

weather at the start of the race with the temperature around 29 degrees Celsius (85 degrees Fahrenheit) which was warm compared to what we were expecting. Little did I know that it would be snowing at the top of the mountain and I would just be wearing shorts and a short-sleeved shirt. At the start we met Arlene Pieper who was the first women to complete Pikes Peak in 1958. In doing this she finished a marathon well before Katherine Switzer ran the Boston Marathon as an officially registered competitor in 1967. The first unofficial woman competitor in the Boston Marathon was in 1966. Unlike Boston, the Pikes Peak Marathon never actually barred women from running the races. When the marathon began in the mid-1950s, women had been running official races up the 13-mile trail to the top since 1936.

What was interesting about Arlene Piper's first Pikes Peak marathon was that her nine-year-old daughter, Kathy Pieper, ran with her to the top of the Ascent. She had originally set out to accompany her mother part of the way but ran all the way to the top and did pass many men along the way. She reached the top in five hours, 44 minutes. At 7 am we got the starting gun. I headed through town towards the forest and the mountains. Maria was slightly injured on the day with hip pain but still wanted to run so she suggested we run at our own pace. If she felt too much pain, she would stop and return to the starting point. There were also cut-off points along the way which may stop her from continuing anyway.

The first part of the run was steep. I clearly remember running for what seemed like a very long time with the upward trajectory and at that point I saw to my dismay a sign that stated only three miles. I thought then that this could be a long day.

The race was very well supported with volunteers at the aid stations which had names like Incline (4.5 km / 2.8 mile), No Name (6.9 km / 4.3 mile), and Bob's Road (8.5 km / 5.3mile). I understand that not just the runners came from all over the US every year to be a part of this event but so did some of the volunteers. I stopped at many points along the way to look over the magnificent view over the high plain below. I wanted to enjoy the run as well as have a go at this tough race.

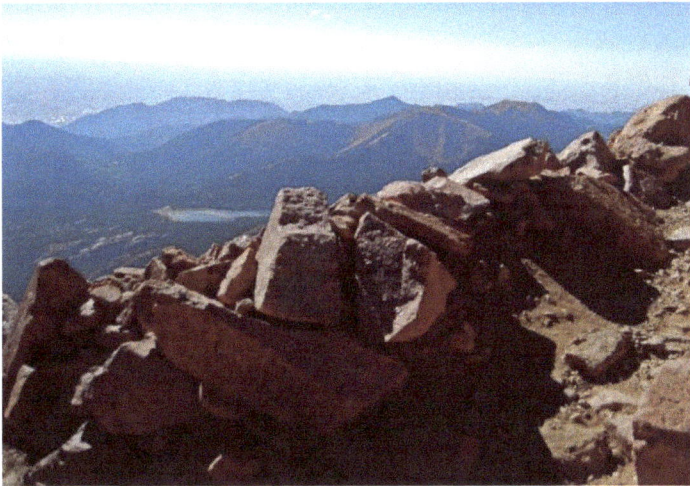

The view on the way up Pikes Peak — The trail is in the foreground

My aim was to get to the top under four hours and back down in just over two hours so a round trip of approximately six and a half hours. I wasn't acclimatised for this type of running over difficult trails at altitude nor running down steep, boulder strewn dangerous mountainous trails, so hopefully my times were realistic. As I passed the tree line at the A-Frame aid station (19 km / 11.8 mile) at around 12 000 feet, I was starting to run short of breath and oscillating between slow running and fast walking.

Once I passed the tree line, the first of the lead runners ran past. I marvelled at how they could run so fast on such challenging terrain and in such conditions. Touru Miyihara was the first runner to pass then Alex Nichols and Jason Delaney. When I ran onto the 'golden staircase' (19.5 km / 12.2 miles) which was the final stretch to the summit there was a line of runners slowly tramping to the top crisscrossing back and forth across the cold forbidding landscape. There was a rough path and, as people were now coming down, it was challenging to keep going up, to avoid the large boulders and pass runners while out of breath. Breathing was the hardest part of all. I finally reached the top just over my four-hour target and a volunteer gently touched me on the shoulders and pointed me back down the mountain. He didn't want anyone staying up there for too long as it was cold and snowing, and with the exertion and lack of oxygen it was exhausting.

Incredibly, I felt with each step downward more and more refreshed. It was the increasing amount of oxygen I was getting. Quickly I was recovering, feeling better and more energised. I ran down the trail at a reasonable but increasing pace. A few faster runners passed as I was still cautious on the dangerous terrain. Some of the runners mentioned the technical nature of the descent which I figured to mean the challenge of the trail, the descent, and the obstacles.

At this point just above the tree line I passed Maria and was filled with pride for her. She was injured, probably from a muscle strain in her hip, but she didn't give up. Onwards she trudged well ahead of other runners and the cut-off times. I knew she was in pain, but she was determined to finish. I think she was just taking one step at a time. When she was two kilometres from the summit, above the tree line, she was struggling, gasping for breath and at one point on her knees vomiting. Such were the extreme conditions. She was approached by a first aid officer, but she refused to exit the race as she knew shortly she would be at the top and then heading downwards. When she reached the summit, the volunteers wanted her to stop again as she was in pain with tears in her eyes but quickly, she turned downward to finish the marathon. She figured there was no point entering a marathon if she didn't finish it and no point having a discussion with an official at this point in the race.

When I passed the A Frame aid station (24 km / 15

mile), I was feeling much better and lengthened my stride. Unfortunately, rocks seemed to jump out at me, and tree roots were higher than I was lifting my foot. On more than one occasion I tripped and slid among the rocks and boulders. Luckily, I just had bleeding knees and palms but no serious damage. Still I lifted my pace as the trail became better with fewer obstacles. At this stage of the race there were also fewer runners about. I often ran alone.

At the No Name aid station (35 km / 22 mile), I lengthened my stride as we entered the forest only to trip on a tree root and slide along the gravelled path for what felt like a few metres. I lost more skin from my knees and my hands as I tried to stop the slide on the path which was covered in gravel. I lost a bit of my pride with it, but then I rationalised that running the Pikes Peak Marathon was supposed to be challenging so having blood running down my shins and splattered on my shirt was fitting. The temperature was rising. After freezing temperatures at the summit, it was now over 32 degrees Celsius (90+ degrees Fahrenheit) in the last few kilometres. I was feeling comfortable, so I picked up my pace. The rocky path had turned smoother under the trees and it was like being back in Singapore again with sweat running down my back and face and washing some of the blood from my legs.

As I raced out of the forest onto the road in Manitou Springs, I knew the finishing line wasn't far away. I cruised down the road over the finishing line feeling elated with a time of just over six and a half hours. To be honest I have never cruised over a finish line. Whether it was a short 5-kilometre race or a 56-kilometre ultramarathon I always gave my best and typically was exhausted at the finish but in most cases would then recover well.

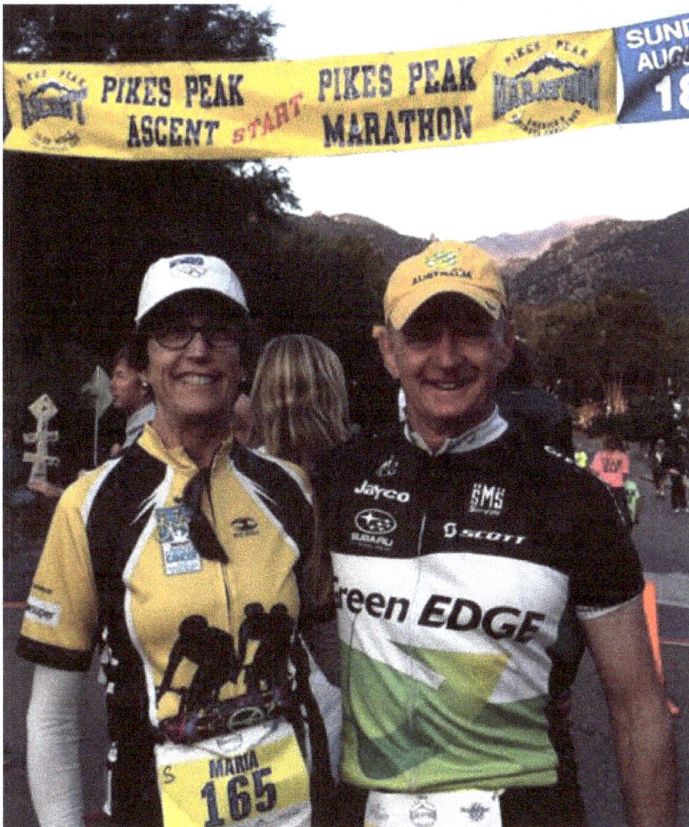

Maria and Michael — Pikes Peak Marathon

Maria came in later, feeling exhausted but still elated that she finished in a reasonable time and under the cut-off. Many people didn't finish. Running accidents occur on that mountain and people in the past have died during the race. It was that sort of event.

> *'No matter how slow you go, you are still lapping everyone who is on the couch.'*
> *– Anonymous*

Chapter 15

Standing in a ski shop – being positive

What does an advanced cancer diagnosis and a ski shop have in common?

Montréal's Marathon in September is run as part of the 'Rock 'N' Roll' series. LikeLA, Seattle and later Denver, the race is run to the accompaniment of bands along the route, real bands, not just music. There were two dozen live bands on the course that weave through the city and neighbourhoods. It really adds to the excitement and entertainment of the runners and the spectators. The Montréal Marathon is a running festival like many major races these days with five different races. There is a 1-km run for kids, 5-km, 10-km, the half-marathon (21.1 km) and the main marathon (42.2 km).

The city is the most populous in the Canadian province of Quebec and the second- most populous city in Canada. It has a population of approximately 1.9 million people including some suburban areas. The broader metropolitan area has a population of approximately 4.1 million. I needed to be in Montréal in September for a conference, so we checked up on whether there were races on at that time. Fortunately, the Montréal Marathon was on the weekend before the conference, so we registered for the run. After the Pikes Peak Marathon, we felt good and as the weather was moving out of summer into autumn, we had a good summer's training behind us and felt not only good in spirits but fit as well.

The Canadians are wonderful people and Canada must be a nice place to live. Montréal, because of its cultural diversity, is considered to be the cultural capital of Canada and is Canada's centre for French-language television productions, radio, theatre, film, multimedia, and print publishing. It also has a tradition of producing both jazz and rock music.

Because of my travel commitments, our visit to Montréal involved a short stay around the business conference so we arrived on the Friday night and ran the marathon on the Sunday. There was little time to acclimatise or take in many tourist attractions. We did walk up beautiful Mont Royale which overlooked the city with Little Italy on one side and the St Lawrence River on the other. The weather was getting cooler but after the Pikes Peak race that was welcome. Autumn is normally pleasantly mild in Montréal. Snow is rare before November as is a heat wave, so we were expecting ideal running conditions. On one business trip when I was in Montréal it was -38 degrees Celsius (-36 degrees Fahrenheit) so I knew it could get very cold.

The race went well, and we ran together. The pace was on schedule and we were hoping for a new PB and BQ. That was not to be, however, as we weren't able to keep the fast pace over the last five kilometres. We came in with BQ times just a few minutes outside our personal bests. Despite this, Maria won her age group and was presented with a beautiful plaque as the fastest woman in her category by the organisers of the race, 'Championne Femmes' de Montréal Marathon.

The previous winter which was our first in Colorado, involved us settling into work and life in a new city, state, and country. We have some friends, Harold and Debbie, who lived in Breckenridge. They kindly invited us to stay with them in one of the ski areas. Being from Australia and recently Singapore we hadn't had the opportunity to visit any ski fields in winter let alone learn to ski. Both Harold and Debbie recommended that we try, so we organised a weekend to stay with them and Harold would take us up to the mountain and arrange ski lessons for a weekend. Harold and Debbie are both accomplished skiers. Harold was also a volunteer mountain ambassador on the Breckenridge ski field. For novices who were learning to ski in their mid-fifties we found the weekend of ski lessons exhilarating and frightening at the same time. Standing on skis looking down a ski slope can be daunting for a novice. On reflection many years later, I realised that initial ski slope was short and almost flat but at the time it appeared so steep Maria took off her skis and walked down it. It was the only chance we had to ski that winter, but we were determined to learn to ski the following season which normally started after Thanksgiving in November and ran until Easter in April.

We planned to try to ski on one day each weekend as the trip from home to the ski areas took only 90 minutes. We could leave at 7.30 and be on the first lift. We could then finish and be back home by 6 pm. To do this properly, Harold recommended we buy our own ski boots and peripheral equipment like ski poles and ski pants. We could always hire skis and purchase some later if we wished. We had good cold weather clothes from our time in Antarctica. We eventually decided not to buy skis at that time and rent them instead.

So, we went down to the ski shop in Denver to look for this ski equipment over one weekend. Prior to this Maria was still having trouble with her hip. The pain was causing continuous problems. We thought it may have been a strain or a small tear in the muscle, but it was persistent and didn't seem to heal. Finally, she went to the doctor and had a series of tests. While we were standing in ski boots for five minutes to see if they're comfortable, she took a telephone call. It was her doctor. He calmly told her that the Magnetic Resonance Imaging (MRI) scan she had done recently indicated that she had advanced secondary cancer in her thigh around her femur and that the cancer was large and well advanced. He speculated that this cancer had metastasised from a primary cancer. Metastases most commonly develop when cancer cells break away from the main tumour and enter the bloodstream or lymphatic system. This means that the cancer cells can travel far from the original tumour and form new tumours when they settle and grow in a different part of the body.

But Maria didn't have a primary cancer from which to get a secondary cancer. She queried the doctor and he recommended she come into the surgery immediately to discuss it with him and that she should get some more tests done. As we stood there in the ski shop trying to process this horrible news we were just given, all sorts of terrible things came to mind. The words secondary, large, and advanced seemed too hard, scary, and painful to think about. When the shop attendant came over to ask about the ski boots, he could see Maria had tears in her eyes, so he quietly moved away. We agreed that we should go to the doctor immediately but what about the ski boots? As it was our nature, we decided that we needed to stay positive and buy the boots. Things would work out and we would get to use the boots together sometime in the future.

The visit to the doctor went badly. He confirmed what the specialist said who reviewed the MRI images and clearly believed that the image around her femur was an advanced secondary cancer. He recommended more tests followed by a visit to a specialist surgeon with the test results. Maria explained that she did have the pain before the recent marathon but there didn't seem to be a link with the marathon as the specialist's conclusions were clear. We were advised that the specialist was very, very experienced. The additional tests were completed and followed by several weeks of torment and anguish as you could expect with the diagnosis that we received. I really feel for people who go through this hell. There are tears, anguish, fear, dreadful times sitting in hospital waiting rooms and comments of 'why me' plus the agonising wait. I think the waiting is the worst. Both of our fathers died from cancer plus my sister had recently gone through breast cancer and survived, so we knew the process and what may lie ahead. Surgery, more surgery, chemotherapy, radio therapy, medication, healing, probably the loss of a leg, learning to walk again, recovery and the fear that the cancer would reappear.

Finally, the visit to the specialist was scheduled together with all the additional test results. The specialist and his advisors looked at all the data in the reports and concluded that the MRI interpretation was probably in error and it was most probably a stress fracture in her femur coupled with trauma around that fracture from running the marathon. So, he believed that there was neither a primary nor secondary cancer, just trauma around the pain site! The X-rays showed a stress fracture in her femur which was obscured in the MRI with the bruising from the marathon. Maria and I were concerned with the words 'most probably' and 'maybe' and asked how this could be confirmed. Subsequently Maria went into hospital for a needle biopsy of her femur.

The results confirmed what the specialist advised. She did, however, have osteoporosis and low bone density which was causing the stress fractures in her feet and femur over the past four years. This would require medication in the form of vitamin D and calcium tablets plus other special osteoporosis medication. It's not in us to be angry or bitter. We try to be positive and energetic people, so we thanked the doctors for their advice and wanted to move on with our lives.

It was an enormous relief that the cancer was not there but meant that she would be back on crutches for a time while the stress fracture healed. It also meant she needed to go on bone strengthening medication. So here we were with the relief of the new diagnosis, but this effectively meant the loss of Maria's marathon running career. When you put so much effort into running and receive from it so much joy and have so many amazing experiences it's traumatic to have that taken away, but this paled in comparison to the wonderful news that Maria was cancer free. So many people don't get this positive diagnosis, so we considered ourselves lucky.

She had a BQ time in her hand but no Boston marathon to run. I didn't feel like running the race without her, so we didn't use our BQ times to apply for next year's Boston marathon. The race we always had on our mind was slipping away. We did get to use our ski boots after all, and Maria cautiously learned to ski slowly and carefully as a fall would mean more bone fractures. Again, the words came to us 'baby steps' but in a different context. When we went to Phidippides track training the following week, Maria came on crutches to say hello to all our friends and tell them the news. One runner said to the whole group 'Maria is amazing and brave beyond belief. She ran a marathon with her broken leg and probably did the Pikes Peak marathon with a broken leg as well. What a hero'. I thought the same as well, especially when I remember passing her high up on the Pike's Peak mountain when she was determinedly running ever upwards.

'When something bad happens, you have three choices:
You can either let it define you, let it destroy you,
or let it strengthen you.'
– Anonymous

The following year was a slow one for us runningwise. We were loving life in Denver and in the US. We still ran the five-kilometre races with the Rocky Mountain Running Club and did the Phidippides track training sessions, but for the first time in ten years no marathons were scheduled. Maria kept her running to a minimum after her leg healed. She kept fit and took more interest in cycling as it would put less pressure on her legs.

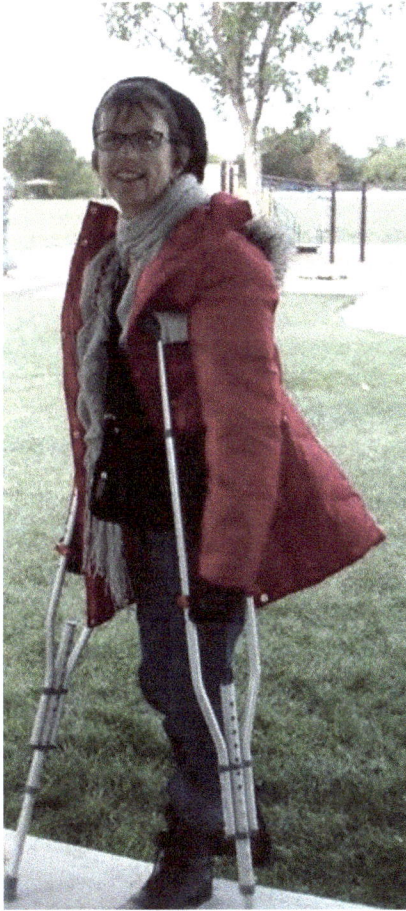

Maria — on crutches again — Denver

Later we joined two friends, Dave, and Deb in the Denver Trail Runners' Club. This group met each Sunday morning on the Rocky Mountain front-range and ran trails up in the mountains. I loved trail running with the fresh air and open spaces. Spring was also very special with all the colourful wildflowers spreading like a multicoloured blanket before us. Maria was less enthusiastic as she was concerned with the distances we ran and the potential for another stress fracture. Sometimes she would stay at home and I would go out with them. Many of the people in the Denver Trail runners also participated in ultramarathons. There are many ultramarathons in the US and the people I was running with were mostly training for an ultramarathon or two over the warmer months of the year.

One event that the runners were entering was the Leadville Trail 100-mile run. This is an ultramarathon held annually on rugged trails and dirt roads near Leadville, Colorado high up in the Rocky mountains. It was first run in 1983 and the route climbs and descends 4800 metres (15 600 feet) with elevations ranging from 2800–3850 metres (9200–12 620 feet). I understood that normally only half of the participants complete the race within the 30-hour time limit.

Another race is the Run Rabbit Run 50- and 100-mile race that runs through the beautiful mountains of the Routt National Forest of northern Colorado up in the Rocky Mountains. The 50-mile race starts at the Steamboat Springs ski area (elevation, 2100 metres / 6900 feet) and proceeds up and across the Continental Divide to Rabbit Ears Mountain (elevation, 3200 metres / 10 500 feet) before heading back and down to the ski area. The 100-mile course starts at the ski area and encompasses Buffalo Pass (elevation, 3200 metres / 10 300 feet) and

Emerald Mountain and back to the ski area. The 50-mile course has nearly 2800 metres / 9000 feet of climbing. The 100-mile course has had approximately 6500 metres / 21 000 feet of climbing.

> *'Trail running makes me feel most alive.'*
> *– Anonymous*

The runners who do these runs are determined and hardy people. So, our runs on a Sunday morning were typically long and involved running trails up in the mountains. One morning we were running in winter and the trail was leading us up a mountain path. I was feeling strong that winter morning, so I ran ahead on my own. As I ran ahead stepping through the fresh snow on the ground, I noticed animal footprints in the snow along the path ahead of me. The footprints in the snow were large. This was a nature reserve, so the prints were not of a cow or horse but something smaller but still something substantial. As I was 300 metres ahead of the other runners, I was alone on this still winter morning and I started looking around at the forest to see if I could see what made the footprints. I felt the trees closing in on me. Was I being watched? My thoughts turned to the mountain lion.

The mountain lion is the second-heaviest cat in the Americas after the Jaguar and can be 0.8 metre (30 inches) in height at the shoulder, and approximately

2.4 metres (8 feet) long from nose to tail. They can jump horizontally around 7–8 metres (23 feet). It's solitary and mostly nocturnal although daytime sightings do occur and they're present in the Rocky Mountains. I knew that it was an ambush predator and in some cases have attacked humans. Over the last 100 years 125 attacks have occurred of which 27 have been fatal. In the general area that we were running in, three fatalities had occurred in the 1990s. An 18-year-old high school student was killed and eaten while jogging a hill above Idaho Springs, Colorado. A 10-year-old boy was killed by an adult female in Colorado's Rocky Mountain National Park while hiking when he got ahead of his family and a 3-year-old boy disappeared after he ran ahead of his father's hiking group in Rocky Mountain National Park. He was never found.

In response to these thoughts I stopped and waited for the others to catch up. When they arrived, I showed them the footprints and one runner simply said 'Yep. Those are mountain lion, all right. He's probably been watching you for a while now. We better stick together.' And that was that. Matter of fact. We kept going. Remember, 'no excuses'!

That winter was also one for extreme weather conditions. In January that year over twenty states from the Midwest to the Southeast and Northeast shivered from what was called a polar vortex. It was a rush of cold air blowing southward from the Arctic plunging many areas into a deep freeze of record low temperatures. As we were in Denver, we experienced this phenomenon firsthand. Temperatures plunged to -26 degrees Celsius (-15 Fahrenheit) one evening. As I had been out running early on most Sunday mornings in the very cold, when the polar vortex hit, I decided it was so cold that I should go out for a run just to experience it. Australians don't get the opportunity to do this very often. So, I dressed up with thermals, Gore-tex jacket and balaclava and went out for that run. I thought that if I waited around for perfect conditions I would never get to run. As most cold weather runners would know once you get warmed up you quickly find you are overdressed. I became so hot I took off the balaclava. The jacket stayed on, however, as I recalled the problem Maria experienced in Antarctica with hypothermia from taking off her jacket after feeling comfortably warm from the running.

One of our friends in the running club did recommend to me to run the Indian Creek Fifties. The races are organised by Human Potential LLC (HPRS) which is committed to bettering and expanding the ultra-running community. HPRS is best known for its winter Fat Ass Series and the Indian Creek Fifties was part of that. I never really understood why it was called the Fat Ass Series and when I checked I found out that it was formed by a group of ultramarathon trail running enthusiasts who have been traditionally known to operate under the moniker of: 'No Fees. No Awards. No Aid. No Wimps.'

The original runners were cowmen so that may be the link with Fat Ass. The original events were 'low-key,' only offering three aid stations, and runners relying on drop bags and a skeleton crew. The moniker changed to no entry fee, no shirts, no medals, no wimps. When I saw this, I liked the idea of a challenging, long, trail race in the mountains with no special treats. You started in the dark and needed to carry your own water. One friend told me he read that the Fat Ass series was trophy running at its worst.

The Indian Creek Fifties are trail races of 50 kilometres (31 miles) and 50 miles and run in the challenging, little used terrain just southwest of the Denver Metropolitan area. The races start in the dark amongst the forest, so runners need head lamps to start and run in the pre-dawn. The first loop climbed to 2438 metres (8000 feet), and quickly dropped down into the Grand Valley as the sun rose and filled the valley with the first rays of light for a few kilometres. The second loop led onto some lovely trails and loop three was through the Roxborough State Park with aspen groves and pine stands. As I had run marathons for over ten years now, I decided to run this ultramarathon trail race for I had at least one marathon in the year. I completed it and the 50 kilometres (31 miles) turned out to be 56 kilometres (35 miles). I didn't mind the extra distance as it was exhilarating to run through the forest in the dark just before dawn using a head lamp and to experience running in such wilderness in the

Rocky Mountains front-range area with some friends. The organisers said we were lucky as we got an extra 6 kilometres (4 miles) for free! The only problem was that I ran out of water with 4 kilometres (3 miles) to go and became very dehydrated. Lucky for me my friend stopped on the way past and gave me some water. I remembered 'no aid and no wimps'. I should've taken on more water in the Camelbak I was carrying on my back.

Overall, I liked the camaraderie of the trail runners. They're great people who love running challenging distances in difficult environments. One female trail runner said, 'It was so cold one morning on one of the trails that some of the water in my drink bottle froze'.

Cold weather running — 'It is only cold
if you are standing still.'
— Anonymous

Chapter 16

The race that never was

We were standing beside the road. It was cold and dark in pre-dawn on the edge of the Rocky Mountains. We were high up and overlooking the high plain before us to the east with the city of Denver down below in the distance. The city's glittering streetlights outlined the geometric design of the city. The city was still asleep. It was that early. The thousand or so runners beside us lined the road up and down in the dark. We could just make out the shadowy people in the distance. We were waiting patiently. Waiting for the race.

A few years before this, when I first drove past Boulder, Colorado, I went up into the foothills. It was a Sunday, and I was amazed by the number of cyclists going out for a ride pedalling higher and higher up into the mountains. On one trip through the high Rocky Mountain National Park up near Estes Park we passed a cyclist on the Trail Ridge Road at 3650 metres (12 000 feet). Why was a cyclist up there? It was high up, the road climbs were steep, the declines were steep and dangerous plus the oxygen in each breath was much lower compared to sea level. I asked some colleagues, and the reply was longer than I expected. There are the three main university towns along the foothills, Golden, Boulder and Fort Collins. The universities were Colorado School of Mines, The University of Colorado, and Colorado State University respectively in those cities and the people I saw were probably students and/or athletes training at altitude to get fitter and faster. Many students move to these universities at the graduate and post graduate level to study and compete in college level athletics. In addition to that, the US Olympic & Paralympic committee is headquartered in Colorado Springs, which is just south of Denver, once again in the Rocky Mountain foothills. I now realised that we were living surrounded by very high quality if not elite training facilities for the US Olympians, aspiring US Olympic athletes, and professional athletes.

It took us a while to get used to the altitude in Denver. It's called the mile-high city because it is in the centre of the Front Range Urban Corridor between the Rocky Mountains to the west and the High Plains to the east at 1560–1730 metres (5130 –5690 feet). When I first arrived, I walked briskly up four flights of stairs at the office and had to stop at the top as I was short of breath and felt like I was having a seizure. I was fit but it still caught me by surprise. Initially we took our running training carefully but quickly we got acclimatised. Training and racing at that altitude became normal.

We looked at doing some high-altitude half-marathon races to help with our training. It seems strange that we would consider a half-marathon race as a training run, but we essentially did a half-marathon each weekend in training so doing that length of a race was normal. In that region there were some famous half-marathons. Some were up in the mountains like Estes Park near the entrance of the Rocky Mountain National Park at 2300 metres (7500 feet) and others started up in the mountains and ran downward like the George Town (2600 metres–8500 feet) to Idaho Springs (2300 metres–7500 feet) half-marathon. In some other locations there are marathons that run downhill all the way. Revel Rockies have a marathon which is described as a fast and beautiful road race which features a smooth downhill slope. It starts at 3200 metres (10 510 feet) and ends at 1770 metres (5800 feet) with a drop of 1430 metres (4700 feet). Some runners do the downhill races to get a PB or even a BQ time.

Under the Boston Athletics' rules running downhill is not cheating, so some runners aim to use these runs to qualify for the Boston marathon. Over thirty years ago in the 1980s British researcher Mervyn Davies conducted treadmill tests that indicated that each one per cent of upgrade slowed elite runners by about 3.3 per cent. This translates to ten seconds per kilometre if someone is running at a five-minute-per-kilometre pace. Over a marathon it calculates to a time approximately seven minutes slower. If the opposite is true, then a five-minute-per-kilometre runner can cut seven minutes off their marathon time. At two per cent it may have twice the effect so the runner would cut fourteen minutes off their time. While this is not as significant as many people would expect, it can still be the difference between qualifying and not. My view is that running at altitude is challenging compared to running at sea level so while the downhill running is an advantage the high altitude takes away some of the benefit.

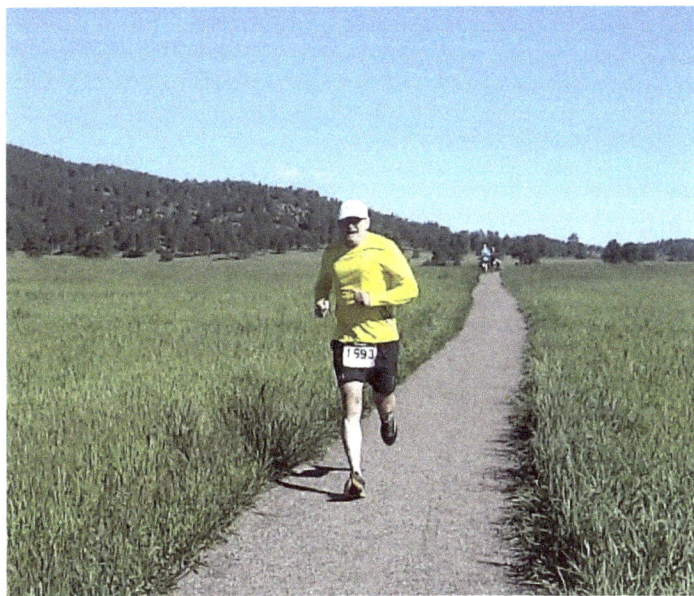

Michael — running in a Colorado Masters Race

Georgetown to Idaho Springs

Our aim was not to run downhill to get a better time but to use the higher altitude races as good training runs. The first high altitude half-marathon we did was the Georgetown to Idaho Springs race. It followed the valley down the mountains on roads and paths alongside the I70 highway which is the highway across the Rocky Mountains from Denver to Grand Junction in the west. It was our first downhill race and while it sounded easier it was, in fact, still a tough race as the start was at dawn and it was at 2600 metres (8500 feet). For Australians to put this into context again, the highest mountain in Australia is Mt Kosciuszko at 2228 metres (7310 feet), so we were starting the race over 250 metres higher than Australia's highest mountain. The race finished at the old mining town of Idaho Springs and the great novelty of the race was that the finishers' medal was in the shape of a pan that was used to pan for alluvial gold. This is in recognition of the history of the town when in 1859 prospector George A Jackson discovered alluvial gold at the site of what is now Idaho Springs. It was the first substantial gold discovery in Colorado. We did this annual race twice over two years as it was a favourite of our running friends from the Rocky Mountain Road Runners and Phidippides Track Club.

Another high-altitude half-marathon we did was the Estes Park half-marathon. Estes Park is a town high up in the mountains in Colorado adjacent to the Rocky

Mountain National Park. It's a popular summer resort location due to the beautiful scenery, cool weather in summer, and proximity to the National Park for day trips and hiking. In Estes Park there is a famous landmark called the Stanley Hotel. This stately Victorian mansion was built in 1909 by Freelan Stanley and is perched up on the mountain side giving it marvellous views over the town below, the picturesque valley and Lake Estes. It's believed that the Stanley Hotel inspired the Stephen King Book *The Shining*. Apparently, the author spent a night there in 1974 and the hotel was a bit run down. He and his wife were the only guests there as the staff prepared to close for the winter and while he was wandering the near empty hotel, he thought that it would make an ideal setting for a ghost story. The now famous room is number 217. The movie based on the book was a psychological horror film produced and directed by Stanley Kubrick starring Jack Nicholson.

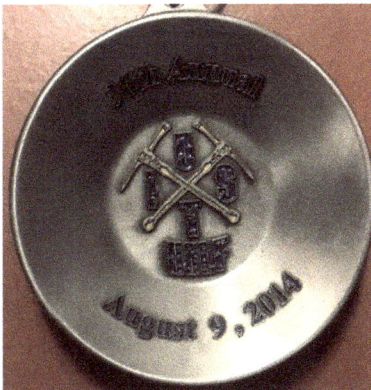

Estes Park

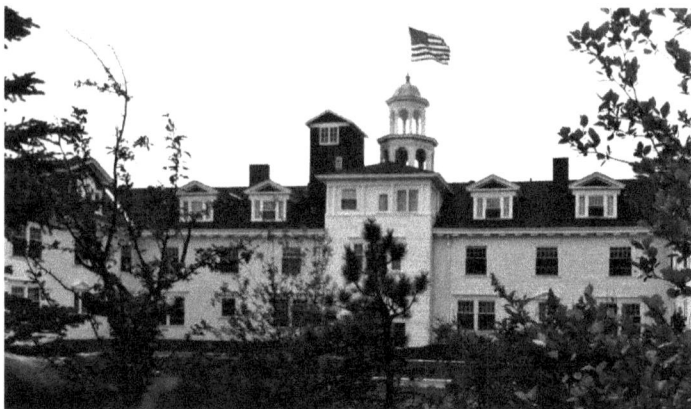

Stanley Hotel — Estes Park, Colorado, USA

The Estes Park Half-Marathon is one of Colorado's most scenic races and one of Forbes top seven most scenic half-marathons. The average elevation is 2290 metres (7522 feet) and apparently it is one of the world's highest paved half-marathons. It's a small race by the number of participants and when we ran it, it was a loop course starting and ending at the local high school, so it wasn't a downhill course. Maria and I drove up to Estes Park a day earlier to give us some time to acclimatise and look around this beautiful town and location. The race went well on the day and as expected we were drained at the end. Despite living in Denver our bodies still found the exertion of running at a much higher altitude a challenge. I came second in my age group which was nice. Maria had recovered from her stress fracture by this time and was taking the runs slowly and getting back to being acclimatised to running at high altitude.

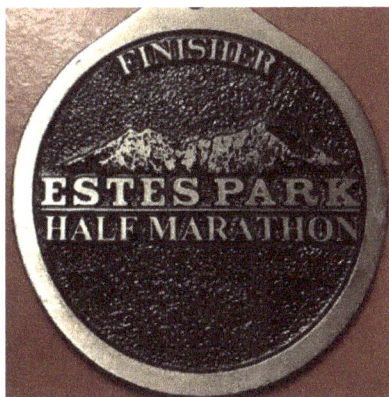

Platte River

In the mile-high city of Denver there were a couple of half-marathons. The key one was the Platte River half-marathon which we did twice. The Platte River is the main river that flows through Denver roughly south to north parallel to the mountains. The race starts in Littleton to the south in the early morning and follows the river northwards past Sheridan, College View, Athmar Park and ends near downtown Denver. The 21.1-kilometre (13-mile) route is essentially on a path that runs beside the river, so it's picturesque. People can run or cycle on the path in normal times but at this time it's full of runners heading north into the city. There are many highlights. One is the party held for runners at the end at which the Breckenridge Brewing Company supplied free beer to the runners! It was a lovely gesture. Even though runners train hard they still enjoy a beer or two in celebration. Breckenridge Brewery started in the mountain town of Breckenridge, Colorado and is the third-oldest craft brewery in the Colorado. The other thing to note is that Maria won a prize in the race which was a meal at the famous Buckhorn Exchange restaurant which is Denver's oldest operating restaurant. It was established 1893 and has occupied the same building for more than 120 years. The interior is stuffed with Western memorabilia and a plethora of mounted animal heads. It's reported that over 500 mounted animals and trophy heads of every description are in the restaurant. It has catered to railroaders, cattlemen, miners, gamblers, businessmen and Indian chiefs. As of 2018, five US presidents have dined at Buckhorn Exchange.

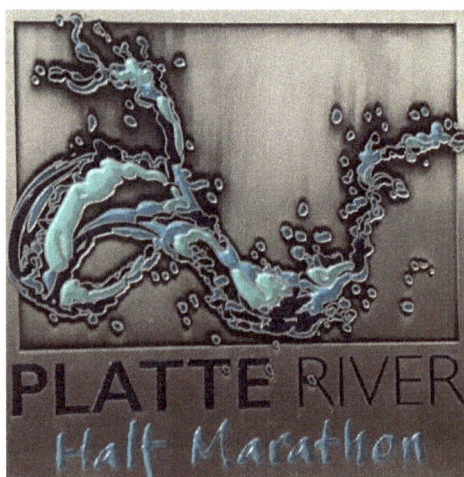

Marathon Training Program — Trailhead Park

The Rocky Mountain Road Runners also held a marathon training run at the Platte River Trailhead Park each year in spring and autumn. It consisted of three well organised races of 16 kilometres (10 miles) and 32 kilometres (20 miles) each to prepare runners for any upcoming marathons. The races consisted of a 16-kilometre out-and-back course which runners could do twice for the full 32 kilometres. It started at the Trailhead Park and ran along the Colorado Front Range Trail, which was a very well maintained, pretty trail by the river with the mountains in the background. As Denver and many of the surrounding towns are old gold mining locations it was not unusual to do this run on a Sunday morning and see people panning for gold in the river. Maria and I did this training series several times and I was also the race director multiple times as well.

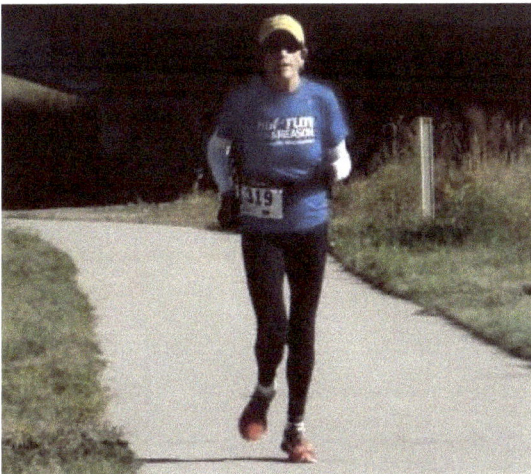

Maria running Trailhead Park

Rocky Mountain Triathlon — Highest Triathlon in the World'

Like many of the events in the US, the race was preceded by the singing of the National Anthem. I love this ritual, and on that day, it was a most memorable one. All the participants were crowded in the cold, early morning light around the start line at the edge of the lake. We were shivering with our bare feet turning pale blue in the cold and the soft soles of my feet hurting from standing on the rocky shoreline.

The announcer checked that the microphone was working, cleared his throat a few times and advised the waiting participants and supporters that the singer was unable to make it that morning because she had laryngitis. There was a lull. I remember hearing a few sighs in the crowd. Some people already had their hand placed over their hearts in anticipation of the anthem. After a pause and recognition of the disappointment in the crowd, the announcer asked if anyone would sing the national anthem.

Almost immediately, a woman triathlon participant, dressed in a long-sleeve black wetsuit with her short dark hair poking out from underneath her distinctive red swimmers' cap started moving through the crowd with her swimming goggles perched on her forehead. She quietly walked up the steps to the temporary stage platform that was set up for the announcements. Her pale bare feet, face and hands with the red cap contrasted strongly against the pitch black of her wetsuit. All eyes turned towards her. She calmly walked across the stage and was handed the microphone. Nobody knew who she was and without any musical accompaniment she began to sing. Her beautiful, passionate soprano voice carried the words of the anthem across the lake and beyond as the crowd stood silent, respectful and in awe. It was truly amazing. And just like that she finished, handed back the microphone and it was back to business. She merged back into the crowd as the race announcer commenced the race countdown.

The course started with a swim in the lake. Snow was still visible on the mountain sides to the north of the lake and the icy cold water was running off the mountain into the lake, so it was cold, bitterly cold. There was no ice on the lake, but it felt like there should have been. If I had seen an iceberg I wouldn't have been surprised.

The morning started off cold even though it was summer because we were high up in the mountains of Colorado. Long sleeve, thick wetsuits were required for the swim which was the first leg of the race. The swim leg was two laps of the elongated lake and when I exited the water, I was cold but warming up. One of the officials asked if I wanted help to remove my wetsuit and I politely declined. When I reached the transition point, I realised my error in declining the offer as it took me a full five minutes of struggling to remove my wetsuit. For some reason it stuck to my skin.

Maybe it was the cold or maybe it was my fatigue from the swim in the icy waters. So much for the slick transition from the swim onto the bike. I was soon, however, on my bike, pedalling down the highway next to the beautiful, famous Blue River to a turnaround point for a return leg back up the valley to the starting point. The reason I call the Blue River famous is that it starts up in the Rocky Mountains feeding off the melting snow and runs all the way across the Rocky Mountains picking up more snow melt along the way and getting bigger and bigger. At Kremmling it joins with the Colorado River which flows across Colorado to the west, exiting the state just past Grand Junction into Nevada and eventually through the Grand Canyon. It's the river that formed the Grand Canyon over millions of years ago.

After the bike leg of the race it was back into the transition point where I stored my bike with haste, removed my cycling shoes, donned my running shoes, and raced onto the running path which was alongside the river. Twenty seconds into the race I realised I had forgotten my cap, but it was too late to go back. I would have to run the risk of sunburn which can occur quickly at this altitude. The running route followed the Blue River in the opposite direction and this time to the east heading through Silverthorne to the highway which separates Silverthorne, Dillon, and Dillon Reservoir. At this point the route was at the maximum elevation at 2780 metres (9120 feet) and turned west back along the river to the finish line. I crossed the finish line in good time, exhausted but well ahead of my age group competitors to win my age group.

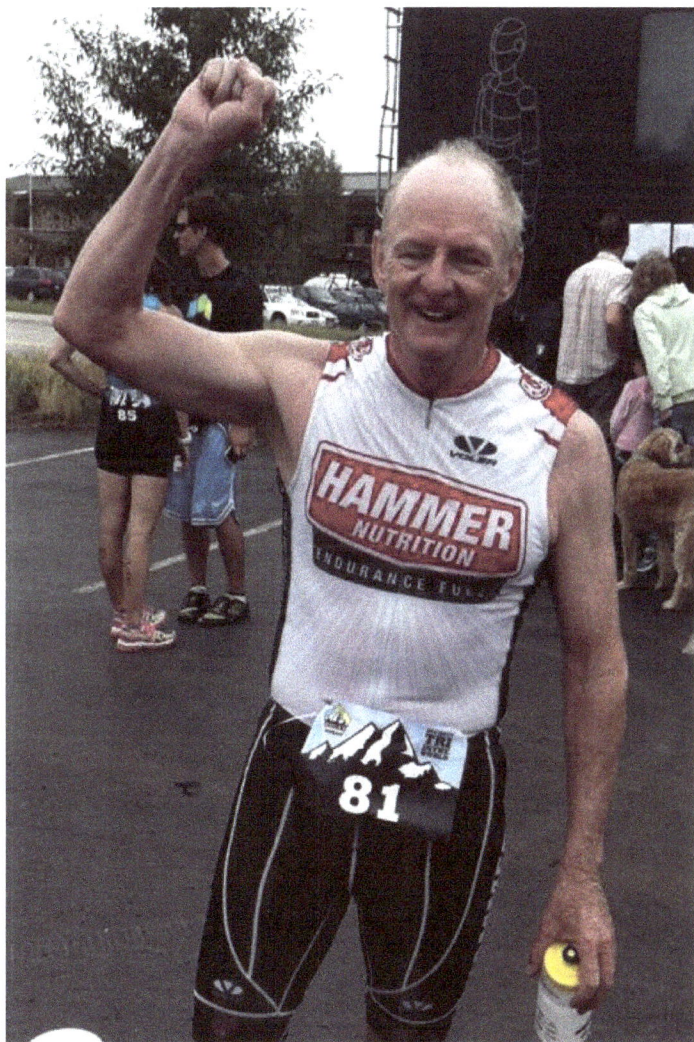

Michael — Rocky Mountain Triathlon — Colorado USA

Revel Rockies

The final half-marathon we entered was the REVEL Rockies Race which was a downhill race in the Rocky Mountains above Denver. There was also a marathon race scheduled for the same day. Many people ran that race to try to get a PB and or a BQ time. The half-marathon starts in a beautiful town called Evergreen at an elevation of about 7410 feet and finishes at 5759 feet in a small town called Morrison which is nearby the famous Red Rocks amphitheatre. The plan for the day was for the half-marathon runners to assemble at a set point and buses would transport the runners to the starting line.

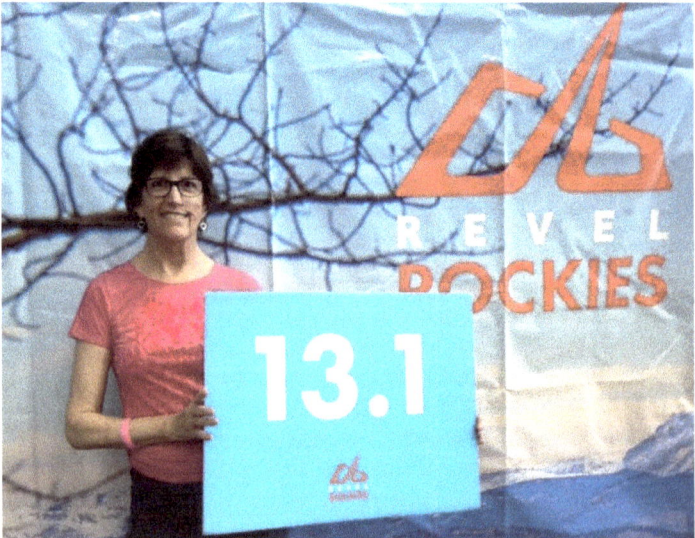

Maria at the Revel Rockies exposition

It was at this point that we were waiting in the dark with a thousand other runners by the side of the road. What happened that day was accurately reported by The Denver Daze's article on July 20, 2015. It read 'REVEL Rockies Race Series Mayhem This Weekend. The Revel Rockies race in Denver this past weekend can be described in three words: confusion, frustration, and miscommunication. The race was cancelled for non-weather reasons, leaving over 1000 participants without transportation to the start line. As the race organizers realized there would not be enough buses for all participants, the decision was made to cancel the half-marathon.' 'Participants had to stand outside for almost two hours in quarter-mile long bus lines with no clear information about the delay.' So, after the two-hour wait on the side of the road the message came through that the race was cancelled and that we should go home! Maria and I called it 'the race that never was'. The race organisers duly apologised and reimbursed the entry fee.

For us it was just another Sunday long training run, but I did feel disappointed for the many who would have trained very hard specifically for this run. Maybe it was their first half-marathon. Maybe they had travelled hundreds of miles to get there only to be turned away.

Chapter 17

Probably the
most famous one of all

As September came around again after the Indian Creek Fifties ultramarathon, so did the Boston Marathon registration process. We had missed out on registration back when we were in Singapore due to our not understanding the process. We didn't use the Boston qualifying marathon times last year because of the Maria's medical scare. We decided as we had qualifying times we should try again to register for Boston. This would probably be our last opportunity due to Maria's propensity for getting stress fractures. The Boston Athletic Association had at the time changed the registration process to provide runners with times better than the qualifying time to register first rather than a first-in basis. Maria's time was around thirty minutes faster than her age group qualifying time and mine was only five minutes faster, so she was able to register first several days before me. When my time came to register, I was hoping that my race time would be sufficient. Finally, it came through and both of us had places in the next year's Boston marathon. Maria felt she had one more marathon in her and as it would be my thirtieth marathon I decided it too would be my last.

Now came the training process over winter. We normally would run at a five minute per kilometre pace (eight minutes per mile) over the 42.2 kilometres. However, Maria didn't want to train up to that level as it would require significant more effort and longer training runs. We decided to train up to a six minute per kilometre level and run the race together at a slower pace so we could enjoy the event more. The concern was her getting another stress fracture as she had already been on crutches three times in the last four years. The six-minute-per-kilometre level was still within the BQ time for Maria's age group.

We were conscious of the recent Boston Marathon bombing, a terrorist attack that occurred on April 15, 2013. At approximately 2.49pm that afternoon, with more than 5600 runners still in the race, two pressure-cooker bombs packed with shrapnel and hidden in backpacks among crowds of spectators lining Boylston Street exploded. It occurred near the finish line. The two bombs killed three spectators and wounded more than 260 other people. It was planned and carried out by two brothers on their own and not connected to any terrorist groups.

We travelled over to Boston and stayed down near the harbour in the Bostonian Hotel. We allowed ourselves a day to acclimatise before the race and check out the famous finish line adjacent to the Boston Common and on Boylston Street outside the Public library between Dartmouth Street and Exeter Street. The finish line is permanently painted on the road and can be easily seen on Google Maps. We visited the pavilion, collected our race numbers and race shirt before catching up with some friends and taking some photographs at the finish line. We took note of where the buses would leave from the following morning to take us to the starting line.

Boston is also a lovely, historical place which we enjoyed visiting. We loved walking across to the Bunker Hill Monument and then down the Charles River past the Massachusetts Institute of Technology to Harvard University. Often rowers would be on that famous river rowing their eights, quad, double or single sculls. As Harvard is such a renowned university we would walk through the grounds before heading across the Anderson Memorial Bridge to the other side of the river and down past Boston University. On the way back to the hotel we would always detour to the Granary Burying Ground, which is the historical cemetery first established in 1660. It's the notable resting place for many Revolutionary War era patriots like Paul Revere and three signers of the Declaration of Independence, Samuel Adams, John Hancock, and Robert Treat Paine.

On the morning of the race I looked up the weather forecast and saw it would feature chilly temperatures, strong gusty winds and developing rain showers. The winter that plagued Boston with record-setting snowfall had not gone yet and unseasonably cold temperatures, rain and wind from a storm system were moving through the area. Through the morning the temperatures were expected to be in the four to nine degrees Celsius (40s Fahrenheit) range only changing a few degrees. Rain was expected. Winds were expected to increase and could gust to near 50 kilometres per hour (30 mph). So, the weather though unpleasant, was nothing we hadn't experienced before. It would've been nice to be sunny, warm and still with blue skies but that was not to be. We got up early and arrived in plenty of time for the bus which took us on the journey to Hopkinton, Massachusetts, the starting line.

As I sat on the bus, memories of the last twenty-nine marathons came rushing back. I saw flashes of my first marathon on Rottnest Island which I ran with Steve many years ago, then of us standing at the finish line in Antarctica and of Maria standing on the winners' podium in the desert of Egypt. After all our running I still think the Boston Marathon is the most famous, historical, and special marathon in the world. The Two Oceans and Rio de Janeiro are much prettier, the Antarctic colder, the Great Wall more exhausting, Pikes Peak more difficult and extreme, and Singapore hotter and more humid, but Boston was special to us. Every single runner on the course had to earn their way into this race by achieving a challenging qualifying time. There are some charity entrants, but we focused on the runners. We started this journey over ten years ago. We got out of our comfort zone, reached for a target of initially finishing an extreme marathon event and then challenged ourselves again and again to get faster, train harder, and finish more difficult and longer races to get here. We were able to share the race with so many talented runners from around the world who also had to earn their place. We were humbled to be among them and didn't take this experience for granted. My experience is that most people who get involved in strenuous exercise including runners are generally wonderful, humble, positive, and energetic people. It takes effort to get off the couch and run but that's what they do every day.

It was cold, and like in Perth many years ago, we just wore shorts, a yellow Boston running shirt, and our newly acquired Boston runners' cap. It was not just cold, but the rain had started earlier than expected and there was a slow breeze making it seem colder. The runners were leaving in waves, so we needed to wait in the cold under a marquee to keep the rain off until it came our turn. We picked up the large plastic bags that were discarded by the runners who left early and huddled inside them to keep warm. We didn't think to bring along an old sweatshirt which we could discard along the way. Despite all that, the crowds screamed louder as each wave of runners took off. Shortly it was our turn, and we were on our way from Hopkinton towards Boston City. The route in my view was relatively flat especially after the races we had done in the past.

Despite the rain, cold and wind, the spectators lined the whole of the 42.2 kilometres (26.2 miles) which apparently is typical for the run. As we passed kilometre 20, the Wellesley girls were there at the fence giving out kisses to runners despite the weather. The residents had set up tents, fires, and had parties in their front yards. They were very generous giving out pieces of orange, sweets, tissues, and water. When we got to kilometre 30 at the Newton Hills just past the Newton fire station, I saw the first of the hills. After all that we had run through over the past years, coupled with the slower than normal pace we were running at, we passed over the hills easily. Having the people of Boston cheer us on helped carry us along.

Heartbreak Hill came and went without a tear, and then we went past Boston College with just 8 kilometres (5 miles) to go. We started passing more and more runners as we were still running with ease at the pace we set, but for many it was the end of the race and they were at the end of their endurance. Then we entered the straight. The finish line loomed in the distance with thousands of spectators lined along both sides of the road. They were roaring with support as each runner came past and over the finish line. To celebrate we ran down the side of the runway giving all the spectators a high five. They cheered and cheered joining in our celebration. We passed the finish line with our hands in the air in celebration of years of training and racing to collect the coveted Boston Marathon medal. It was lovely to finish but we were also aware that it was still cold and wet. We were relieved when some volunteers handed us special Boston Marathon ponchos to keep us warm and dry.

At the finish, we turned around and looked down the final straight at the runners still coming in exhausted but relieved. There were cheers, tears and arms raised in a salute to the finish. That was our last marathon finish line, but it held no regrets, only years of wonderful memories. We were so pleased to finish on such a famous historic, course. We then quickly moved up the street. The recent bombings were on my mind despite the substantial police and security presence. We just didn't want to take any chances, but the security and police along the course did a magnificent job. We felt safe all the way. I was looking forward to the hot shower.

So, our marathon journey was over. We had learned so much, met many wonderful people like Jewel, overcame so many obstacles, seen so many amazing things and places, and had numerous memorable experiences. Maria stood on the winners' podium numerous times in many countries and suffered from hypothermia in Antarctica. We had passed people sitting crying with exhaustion on the Great Wall of China and reached the goal of multiple PBs and BQs while travelling the world. It had taken us to Antarctica to see the beautiful scenery that only a few people get to see in their lifetime. We sat nearby as chinstrap penguins waddled around us and watched orcas chase whales through the Antarctic waters. I had completed thirty marathons, two of which were 56 kilometre races. Maria had completed twenty-four marathons including one ultramarathon. We had run all seven continents and in twenty-two countries and joined the Seven Continents Club. It was a wonder-filled journey. Now it's time to start yet another.

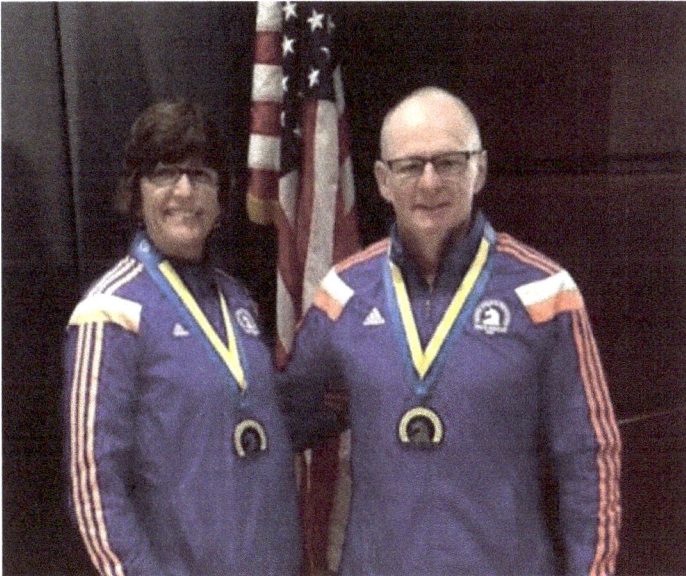

Maria and Michael after finishing the Boston marathon

'I may not have gone where I intended to go, but I think I have ended up where I intended to be.'
— Douglas Adams

Chapter 19

'A candle loses nothing by lighting another candle'

This quote is by James Keller, relates to the fact that when a candle lights another candle it doesn't cost the original candle anything, but the extra candle helps brighten up the room. This can also mean that it doesn't cost us anything to help other people, but it certainly can have a profound impact on their lives and brighten up their day. When I think back to the message from Steve, he didn't need to send it, but he knew that I liked running and he wanted to know if we could do something special together. He was helping me do something exciting. I like the quote from the Dalai Lama, 'When you talk, you are only repeating what you already know. But if you listen, you may learn something new.' He means there's enormous value in listening to what people say to understand and learn.

So is the case with running. Steve shared a message and an idea. I listened, understood, and did something about it. In this case by listening and doing something it had a profound impact on my life, Maria's life, and that of many other people. Some people call it the ripple effect. I also think back to the German tourist I met in Singapore who shared with me his travel philosophies which also led us on many adventures. I wouldn't have done so many amazing things if I chose not to say hello to him that day and if I had not listened.

In 1989 Stephen Covey published a book titled *The 7 Habits of Highly Effective People*. Principally, it's a business and self-help book which I read at the time and took from it many lifelong habits. While I liked many of the chapters I was particularly struck by chapter five entitled 'Seek first to understand, then to be understood'. I thought that it was amazing that a worldwide bestselling author was dedicating an entire chapter essentially to advising people that in order to be successful you need to listen to people to take the time to understand what they're saying. It's from this basis of understanding you can move forward. It also sounds a lot like the Dalai Lama's quote 'But if you listen you may learn something new'.

When I was in my twenties, I did things a certain way based on my family values, training and experiences. Then at around thirty years of age I read a well-known book called *How to Win Friends and Influence People* by Dale Carnegie. Dale was a successful American writer, businessperson, salesperson, and lecturer. The book fascinated me. I read and reread it. It changed my life. Up until then, I didn't realise many things I was doing could have been done much better and that I was not listening to people, really listening to people. The book presented several key themes. My take on the things I learned was to be genuinely interested in others, be a good listener, let other people do a lot of the talking, and try and see things from the other person's point of view.

If I combine these several things from the Dalai Lama, Stephen Covey and Dale Carnegie we arrive at some fascinating common themes which for many is common sense but as someone said to me this week, 'Sometimes common sense is not so common.' Listening and understanding people is an important skill. Learning from what you hear is critical and so is doing something about what you've heard and understood.

So, what does this have to do with running and marathons? Well quite a lot really! You read and hear that staying fit and healthy is important. Nobody wants to be sick or die early. Running, jogging, or walking are easy things to do, low in cost, and combined with a healthy simple diet, can help you live a longer, more vibrant life. So, if you want to keep fit and healthy why not follow a simple healthy diet and go for a run. If people say they're feeling lethargic, unfit, or unhealthy then experience allows us to talk about what we eat and how we exercise. Sharing these experiences to motivate others is like lighting someone else's candle to bring an extra bit of light into their life.

Over time we had coached many people including a

group of runners at interval training in Singapore, been race directors for multiple races in Denver, worked on the board of the Rocky Mountain Road Runners and continue to volunteer for our local Park Run and other clubs in Perth.

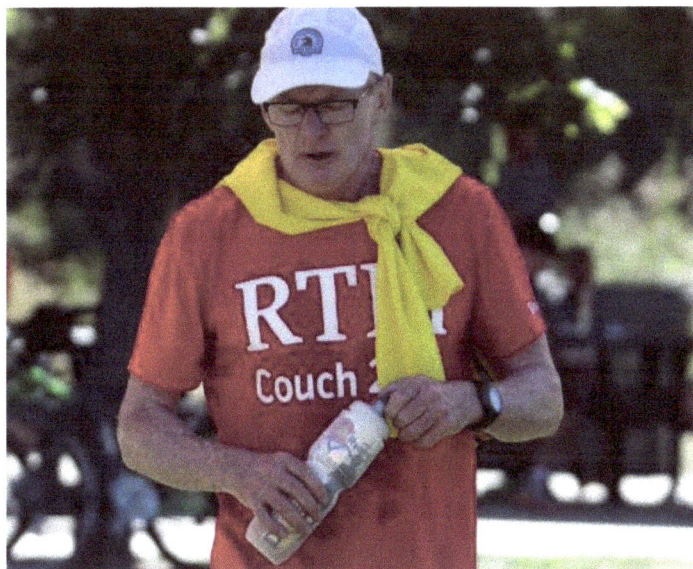

Michael — race director — couch to 5 km program

In our family we all exercise. For some it's running, others cycling or interval training, but we all do it and keep each other motivated. In our final year that we were in Singapore, Maria and I decided to complete an Ironman 70.3, so we asked our son, Aaron, to join us and he did. He moved into training mode and easily completed the event not once but a few years later he completed it again. He has also run many races and cycles several times each week.

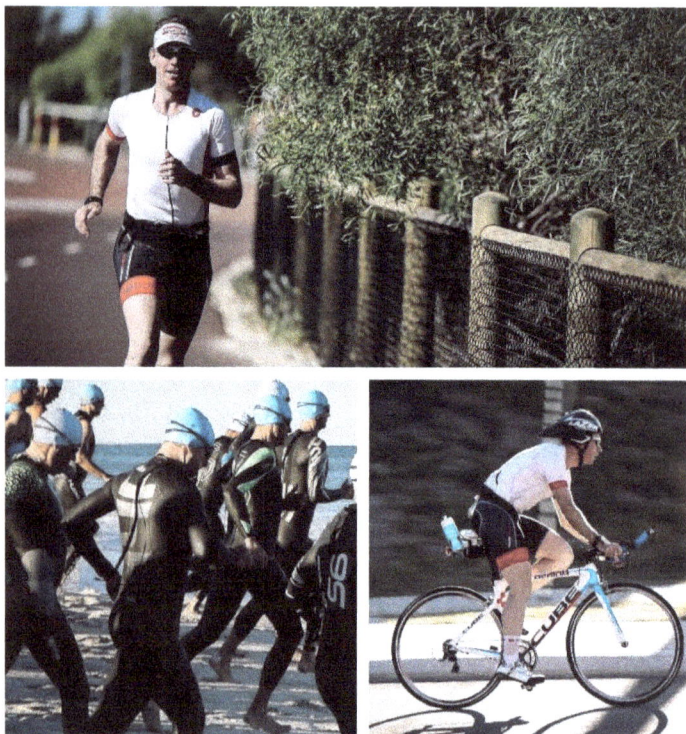

Aaron competing in a triathlon

Our daughter is also into running, swimming, and cycling. Over the past few years, she has completed many road and trail running events, endurance swimming events with her friends, half-marathons and last year for the first time a marathon in Perth. Our other two sons are still very fit and healthy and benefit greatly by the exercise they do. One son, Talbot, has also run a half-marathon with us at an excellent pace of around ninety-six minutes or four-and-a-half-minutes per kilometre. Previously I wrote how I ran an interval training group in Singapore. There are many of these similar groups around the world that help runners for free or at a small cost. A weekly club run is also a good idea as it puts you in a competitive race each week, but the competition is against yourself and your time. I have set out here a few examples of some running groups that we have participated in in various parts of the world.

Parkrun is a good run to do. It was founded by Paul Sinton-Hewitt in 2004 at Bushy Park in London, England. It is now a worldwide network of free 5-kilometre runs which are typically held on a Saturday morning. It can be found at https://www.parkrun.com

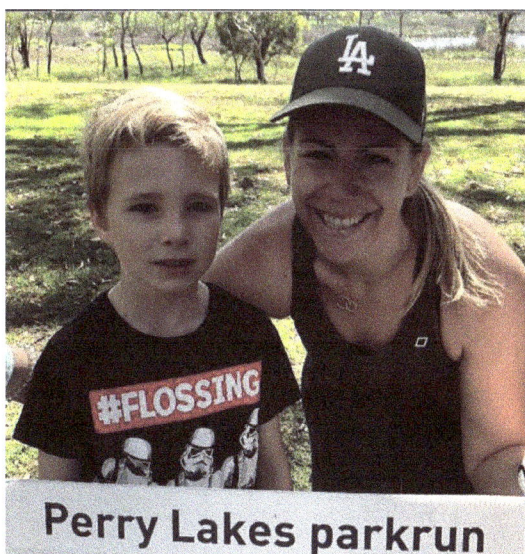

Jason and Frances — Perry Lake Park Run

Perth — West Australia Marathon Club

https://www.wamc.org.au/

The WAMC is a club in Perth that scheduled weekly interval training and races on most weekends ranging from shorter 10-kilometre runs to marathons.

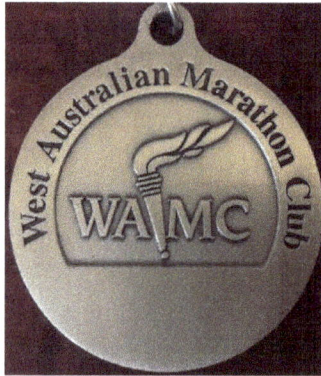

Perth — Perth Masters Athletics. They have weekly road and trail running events http://www.mastersathleticswa.org/

Singapore — MacRitchie Runners 25 — Singapore's Premier Running Club https://mr25.org.sg/

The MacRitchie Reservoir Park in Singapore is a popular spot for exercise enthusiasts. It has hiking trails which the MacRitchie runners regularly use for races and training runs. It is a twelve-hectare green haven bordering the country's first reservoir and the Central Catchment Nature Reserve. The park is also a popular venue for schools and organisations to hold cross-country events, allowing participants to run through designated trails while embracing the wonders of our native biodiversity. Some of the MacRitchie runners also hold interval training every Tuesday evening.

Denver Colorado, USA — Rocky Mountain Road Runners

Maria and I were on the board of the RMRR and they are a great group of people https://www.rmrr.org/

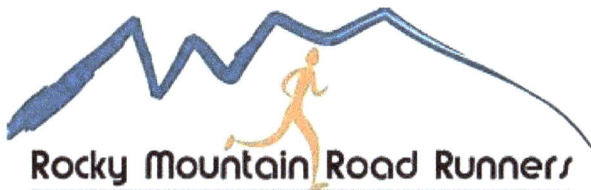

It has just less than 1000 members. RMRR is the club for runners who don't have free time for a weekly meet-up. It was founded in the mid-1950s and RMRR holds monthly runs at varying locations around Denver which are organised to feel like official races. Aid stations are set up throughout the courses, and the starts are staggered. Each event names the fastest female, male, walk group, and since it's highly organised, there is a $35 fee for the full year. The RMRR also hold weekly interval training when the weather is suitable plus marathon training programs at set times during the year.

Denver Colorado, USA — Phidippides Track Club

https://phids.org/

Phidippides Track Club is for those who want to do weekly interval / track training. If you enjoy track training, it's on every Tuesday at 5.45pm, at Belleview Elementary. This club is seasonal from March through October and brings together fast and not- so-fast runners alike. They're a lovely group of people. Maria and I trained with this group for several years.

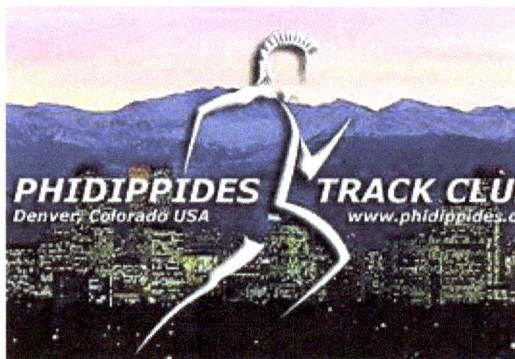

Denver Colorado, USA — Denver Trail Runners

https://www.facebook.com/groups/denvertrailrunners

There are no rules, no sign-ups, or payments to run with this group. Just show up to a Denver Trail Runners session. The group is made up of all kinds of athletes and most of the runs are in the foothills West of Denver, around Morrison, Golden, Evergreen and SW Littleton and sometimes a little further afield. The run is normally on a Sunday morning. Maria and I ran with this group when we lived in Denver.

Denver Colorado, USA — Colorado Masters Running/ Race-walking Association

http://comastersrun.org/

The CMRA is a non-profit all-volunteer organisation that promotes running, race- walking, and fitness by regularly sponsoring distance running-related activities including races, fun runs, training sessions, and social events. Membership and activities are open to people of all ages, abilities, and levels of fitness with awards oriented toward athletes age thirty-five and older.

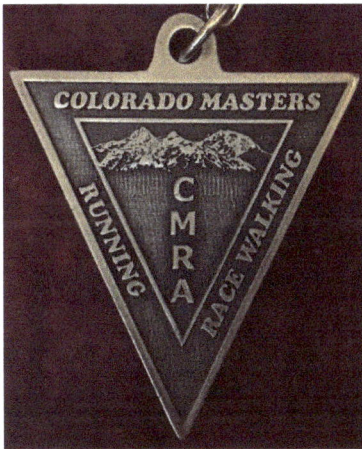

Chapter 20

Shoes, clothes, nutrition, and injuries

I was at the beach on the east coast of Singapore in the early morning. It was light and, as normal, it was still and hot. I was standing in a pair of grey swimming briefs, a coloured swimming cap which designated the division I was in and a pair of swimming goggles. I had done a triathlon before, but this was my first triathlon in Singapore. Two ladies in their twenties were near me. They had on one-piece ladies swimming briefs. We were the odd ones out. It seemed that all the other participants wore expensive, brand-name attire designed for superior performance. Some wore special compression pants and others skin-tight Olympic style swim wear. Nice watches were on their wrists to determine their pace. My wrist felt naked in comparison. I did feel inferior as I thought I hadn't raced here in Singapore before; my torso was bare, and these people were so well equipped. I swallowed back my concerns and even though I had done the training I knew I would try my best. In a triathlon, the swim leg is first, then you run into a transition area, get on your bike, complete the ride, and repeat the transition for the run leg. So, there are three events and two transitions before you run over the finish line.

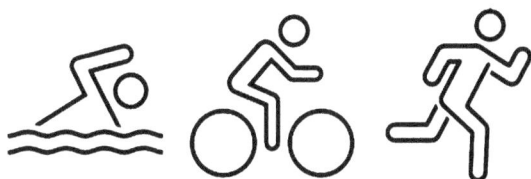

After a few hundred metres into the swim I realised the two ladies and I were leading the pack. With each stroke we inched further ahead. It was a two-lap race around two large buoys out in the sea so after the first lap we did a short run across the sand and back into the water. In this short run I noticed the three of us were ahead of everyone else. This was a surprise to me. Where were the flash, well equipped competitors? At the end of the second lap the three of use exited the water and ran towards the transition point. When I looked back, I couldn't see any other competitors, just some splashes out in the sea. So, I concluded that in the swim leg of the race having fancy expensive racing gear didn't matter at this level. Maybe in elite level races it can create an edge. I was third in the race at this point.

When we went into the bike transition phase I put on a T-shirt, a bike helmet, and shorts. Then I grabbed my bike and ran to the point where I could get on the bike to head out to the bike track. My bike was a $79 bike from the Carrefour. Carrefour is a French multinational corporation that specialises in grocery stores and retail. I knew the bike was nothing flash. I bought it two years before to do the commute from our apartment to karate training so I could warm up for training rather than take a taxi. It was steel, very heavy for a bike with large mountain bike tyres and low-end gears and brakes. As I took off on the bike leg, I noticed everyone else had wonderful, expensive-looking, fast bikes with skinny wheels and multiple gears. Some people had on pointy helmets, aerodynamic sunglasses, solid disc wheels and bikes that resembled a space craft rather than a bicycle. Once again, I did feel inferior. This time it was my bland, inexpensive, large-tyred, heavy, chunky mountain bike. It felt like I was driving a tractor in a Formula-1 race. Although I raced hard to the best of my ability, the other competitors raced past me. When I finished, my place in the race had slipped from third to over 240th. So, I re-entered the transition to drop off my bike and swapped my helmet for a running cap to head out to the run and final leg of the race. This was my favourite part. I raced past the other competitors, picked up over 210 places, and came in 22nd.

I learned from this experience that in the bike leg, equipment really does matter. I hadn't done enough bike training but even so the lighter, much better equipped bikes provided a great advantage. In the run and swim, equipment provided less of an advantage, performance largely depended on training and effort. A triathlon suit that you could swim, ride, and run in is an advantage at it reduces the transition times. Despite these comments, running shoes for a runner are very important and will in my view over the longer term reduce injuries and enhance performance.

I worked out that I have so far run thirty marathons including two ultramarathons, completed ninety 30-kilometre runs and have run at least a total of 25 000 kilometres (15 600 miles) over the ten-year period running marathons. This equates to running across the US about seven and a half times, over six times across Australia and three times between Paris to Vladivostok. That's a lot of distance and a lot of time in running shoes so I've learned a bit about running shoes and I will outline some of my experience.

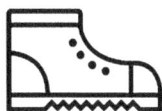

Shoes. If you're just starting out in running, the old shoes you have in the back of the wardrobe for the last fifteen years will not be best for your new running journey. Your shorts, tights, T-shirt and cap will probably be just fine in the beginning, but in running, shoes are important as they can assist performance and, more importantly, reduce the risk of injury. Over the years I have developed a few rules that I stick with when I am buying shoes.

The major brands all put a lot of effort into designing, manufacturing, and improving their shoes. Some websites do regular reviews on the brands and new shoes so please check them out. Here are a few examples: marathonhandbook.com and runnersworld.com

Close-fitting shoes are a trap for the new runner. While you need the shoes to fit well there needs to be at least a thumb space between the longest toe and the end of the shoe. I do this by trying on a shoe that is half-to-one-size too long. If I can press my thumb between the end of the longest toe and the end of the shoe, then it's a good fit for me to run in. The reason for this is that as you run each step and place your foot onto the pavement, the toe moves forward slightly. If the toe hits the end of the shoe repeatedly then you will end up with a bruised toe and potentially lose a toenail. Maria and I have lost many toenails this way. A shoe that works well doing five kilometres may not be good for repeat ten-kilometre runs and so on. So, the shoe needs to be a good fit around the foot but longer in the toe.

I have tried many of the major brands over the years including Brooks, Nike, Asics, Adidas, Saucony, Mizuno, Newton, and New Balance. I like all these brands, but I found that I kept going back to Brooks for running and Saucony for trail runs as they worked for me. They're Jewel's favourites as well. Trail running shoes are different from road running shoes, so we bought different shoes for different surfaces. Maria also used Saucony but used a Merrill shoe in Antarctica. Puma, Hoka and Skechers are also reported to be good. I like the Brooks shoes as I found them comfortable, good value for money, and they lasted well. There was also a Brooks speciality store in Perth which I used. I always bought my shoes from a reputable running store like Brooks, where the assistants are runners. While I had in my mind what I wanted, sometimes the assistants provided valuable advice. I generally had at least two pairs of shoes on the go at any one time and rotated them so if I had any sort of foot or knee pain I would rotate out of that particular shoe. I found that my shoes gradually lost their support. I spoke to a podiatrist to get some advice on this and he pointed to the inside sole of the shoe and said if I saw any stress lines there it indicated that the support was being lost.

Running shoes typically lose their support quicker than many runners realised. I use the rule of thumb that shoes need to be replaced every 500 to 800 kilometres or (300- 500 miles). Many times, I would go longer as the shoes looked almost new when the distance was up. If I was running 50 kilometres a week then the shoes would need to be replaced every ten–sixteen weeks. A friend of ours in Denver wrote the date she purchased a shoe on the outside of the shoe, so she knew exactly how long she had it and when it was due to be replaced. I also like to have two shoes in rotation as I never needed to be concerned about 'running in' a shoe.

For people with over-pronation or under-pronation issues, it's always best to consult a podiatrist as they're the experts. I recall walking into a podiatrist one time and complained about a pain on the inside of my knee. He immediately replied that I was wearing the wrong type of shoe and the shoe I was wearing had a slightly softer sole on the outside of the shoe compared to the inside near the arch and this was causing the pain. So, please consult a podiatrist if you need any professional advice regarding your feet. I would also examine the sole of my running shoe from time to time to see where the wear areas were. When I was running, I tried to land softly and evenly on the front of my foot as this was considered to be the best running action. I was also conscious of my running geometry, so my feet and legs were aligned straight forward and not pointing inwards and outwards. I considered this to apply less stress on my knees, ankles, and hips. I also thought about my posture and tried to keep myself upright rather than leaning forward. Other runners prefer the leaning forward approach.

'The say money cannot buy happiness but I have a receipt for shoes from the running store which tells a whole different story.'
— Anonymous

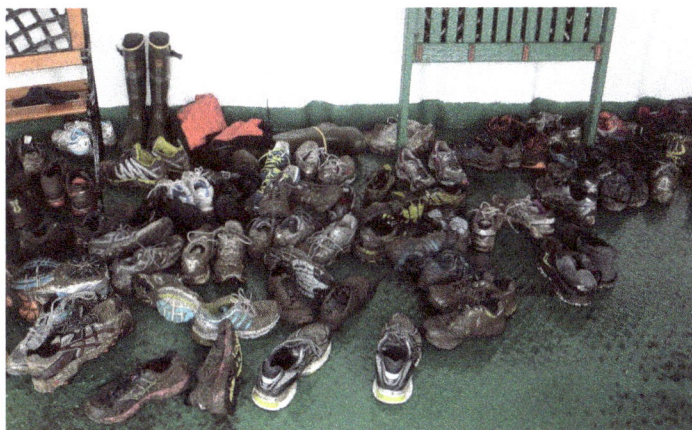

Filthy shoes after the Antarctica marathon

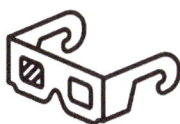

Sunglasses. Many runners always wear sunglasses and the market for fancy, modern-looking, aerodynamic sunglasses for runners is large. There is no real advantage in running with sunglasses as they don't make you run faster, but they are considered by many experts to protect your eyes from glare and sun exposure. They may also help prevent your eyes from drying out from any wind, so they're a personal choice and many runners choose to wear them. Maria won't go out in the sun without them.

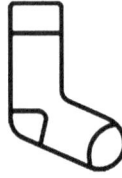

Socks. My choice for running clothing is relatively simple. The area I'm most particular about is socks. Try to imagine a pair of loose socks on your feet inside a shoe. If they crease and fold between your shoe and your foot with each step you take, the fold rubs against your foot. For a short run this isn't a problem. For longer runs I found that old, poorly fitting socks caused blisters on my feet. To counter this, I always used good fitting socks so there were no creases in the socks and no loose bits. On the market now are many excellent running socks which are designed to fit better and stay that way for a long time. For me, better socks are well worth the money.

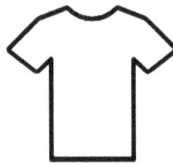

Running shirts. As we spent a lot of time in hot sunny places like Perth and Singapore, I always chose running shirts that cover up the skin well like a lightweight long sleeve running T-shirt. I find cotton T-shirts become very wet, so I normally use a modern moisture wicking running shirt that handles the sweat better. With a moisture wicking shirt, the sweat moves to the outer layer and dries quickly.

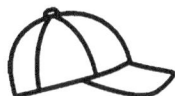

Caps. I always wear a cap and supplement it with sunscreen to prevent sunburn. If you run during the day in hot climates you can get sunburn easily. For someone who is used to running in cooler climates it can be a big surprise where they run in a hot country as they can get very badly sunburnt very quickly, especially in Australia. In Singapore and Perth, I normally tried to run in the evening when the sun wasn't out. If I do choose to wear a short-sleeve T-shirt, I use sunscreen on my arms. In many marathon races they provide all finishers with a souvenir running shirt. I still have many of these and have given away or recycled many more, but these shirts are typically good for running in. One thing worth noting is that for men it's not a good idea to wear a new T-shirt when you run a long training run or a marathon race. The reason for this is that when you are running your T-shirt rubs up and down against your nipples and can cause bleeding. Some people call this nipple chafing. It's a common problem and it's not unusual to stand at a finish line and see men finishing with blood running down the front of their T-shirt. New T-shirts seem to cause this problem more often as older T-shirts seem to be softer on the skin. Some runners apply a layer of Vaseline or put a bandage, like a band aid, over their nipples.

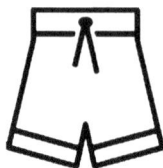

Shorts. I normally run in shorts which are made from moisture-wicking material and designed for running. Some people like longer shorts like basketball shorts, some like shorter shorts, and some like tights. The main consideration for me is that they're comfortable, light, moisture-wicking and don't cause chafing. This comes down to personal choice. I have also used compression shorts. Once again, if you try something like compression shorts and it works for you then use it. There are also compression socks and compression calf coverings. I haven't tried these.

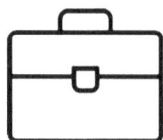

Clothes bag. In marathons the organisers generally provide a secure place to put your carry bag / tote. I use this facility as I can safely store valuables and replacement clothing as it's comfortable to change out of our sweaty clothes into something dry and clean plus warm if it's cold like Boston or Antarctica or hot and steamy like Singapore and Egypt. I have tried using a bumbag (fanny pouch), but I found these incredibly irritating. Running long distance is best done without carrying around odds and ends like keys.

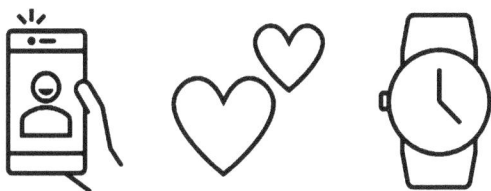

Heart rate monitors. It took me several years but, as I wrote previously, I bought a Pulsar heart rate monitor (HRM) and then a Garmin and I currently have a Samsung smartwatch. Maria has an Apple watch. I like training and racing with a heart rate monitor as I can quickly see how hard I am performing based on my heart rate and pace. In training it also helps me ensure I am training at the correct level to achieve my aims. Having read extensively on the proper use of a HRM I recommend to everyone that it is worthwhile to read up on their use. I still prefer the use of a HRM chest strap rather depending on the wrist measurement as I found my chest strap more accurate. There are lots of brands on the market and I have not used or read up on them all, but my favourite is my Garmin which is now six years old and still works very well.

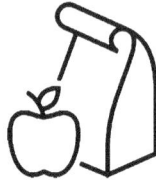

Nutrition during a race. It's common for runners and other endurance athletes to consume some form of food during an event. Some runners strongly believe in carbohydrate loading before an event. In most, if not all marathons, the organisers provide aid stations at set locations with water, a speciality electrolyte drink, and some food. The food can vary as I have seen speciality gels and bars like Shot, Power Bar, Power Gel and Hammer Nutrition but can also include bananas, hot salty potatoes, Mars bars, candy, and oranges. I don't have any special favourite gel or power bar, but I prefer to use Madjool dates for the reasons I mentioned before. I have read widely about food intake during endurance runs and the advice varies from training your body to learn to burn body fat to eating something every twenty minutes. After much trial and error, I took the advice from an Ironman triathlete who was a friend of mine and ate some form of easily digested nutrition every thirty minutes including something immediately before the race. This worked for me and with proper energy intake and electrolyte replacement I found I maintained good energy levels and stopped having cramps.

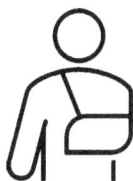

Injuries. Over the time I've run, except for the time I slipped off a small step and sprained my ankle while painting and when I slipped on the trail at Pikes Peak, I've had no injuries. I have lost a few toenails from running in shoes that were poor fitting, but I haven't suffered any significant injuries from running. This isn't the case for many runners. For professional runners they train and race at their maximum so they're much more likely to push their body to and over their limits. They have professional support to help optimise their performance and limit injuries.

I put my injury-free running down to several things.

Firstly, the piece of advice I read very early on was the ten-per cent rule. That's to not increase my running distance by more than ten per cent each week. I felt this gave my body time to adjust to the additional running distance. I think many new runners get injured, exhausted, or disappointed when they start running and try to do too much too soon. Muscles and ligaments that have been not used much for some time and are starting to be used again can get sore or strained. If someone is starting out to run but hasn't run or exercised recently, then the first step is to start walking. A kilometre or mile a day is a good start with two or three rest days a week. Walk with a friend or family member and talk. This makes the time go quickly. Maria and I would do a 30-kilometre (19 mile) run on a Sunday and talk all the way. The distance can then be expanded by ten per cent per week. Once this feels comfortable then a few short runs can be included during the walks. It's good to start with something simple like a short walk and then jog slowly for 50 metres (yards). It may seem like too little, but it enables the body and the person to get used to the new exercise. It's easy to stop exercising when you wake up with sore muscles and feel exhausted but if the slow and steady approach is taken then it gives your body time to adjust. You feel great rather than exhausted and sore.

The second thing we learnt very early on was that if you get injured to stop training and recover. While I have not had any injuries this piece of advice makes sense to me. If you are injured, to continue to train or race can only aggravate the injury and prevent it from healing. When Maria realised, she had stress fractures she stopped running and got professional advice.

The third thing I learned which I believe helps is the concept of cross training. What this means is that if someone is a runner, they could benefit by doing some other exercise to strengthen other parts of the body like the core and upper body muscles. Some of my running friends suffered from weak stomach muscles. While they were excellent and fast runners, stomach muscle issues caused them pain, injury and in several cases required surgery. Some runners also consider stretching exercises like yoga and Pilates to help. I agree with this. For many years, my karate training involved significant stretching exercises to build flexibility and strength in the body. I believed this helped me with running and I continue with this stretching today.

The final thing is I stayed within my limits. I planned to run a maximum of 70 kilometres (44 miles) each week for the weeks prior to a marathon. For a few years I would run up to 80 kilometres (50 miles) a week. This consisted of three 10-kilometre runs, a 20-kilometre run and a 30-kilometre run each week. However, I did not exceed those levels as I was working long hours, travelling and I didn't want to sacrifice my rest days or other activities. Many other runners would easily exceed these levels each week especially a professional runner, but I was comfortable with my training plans and these distances. I also read several articles on interval training and the recommendations were to do interval training once per week. The conclusions from these articles was that more than one session per week could result in injury.

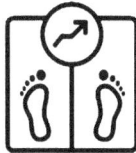

Body Mass. It makes sense that if someone is fit, light in weight and lean then it will be easier for them to run and be an endurance runner than someone who is overweight or obese. I've seen many runners who appear to be significantly overweight and yet they have trained and run marathons, however, they're almost always younger people as it must be easier for a younger person to carry around that extra weight over a race than an older person. As people age, it's easier to continue to run and train if there is less weight to carry around. I have always recommended that people get a medical check-up prior to commencing any exercise to ensure their health is good. The medical professional may suggest ways to optimise someone's weight before commencing the exercise program or combine a weight program with an exercise program.

We have read widely and listened to a lot of people, especially dietitians, I haven't tried any of the fad diets but as I worked in a role that required long hours in the office, very regular international travel and nights in hotels I realised early on that I needed to be watchful of what and how much I ate and drank. During one short six-month period when I first started to travel regularly throughout Asia and particularly to India, I put on over twelve per cent bodyweight. I kept this on for a few years and struggled to get back to my normal weight until a work colleague introduced me to a simple concept which was even publicised at the time, to reduce processed foods plus carbohydrates and consume at each meal a small portion of meat, especially fish, and the remainder would be half vegetables and half fruit.

I continued with this and very quickly my weight went back to normal. This was before taking up running for marathons. The key for me was the reduction in carbohydrates and processed foods as both previously were a base in my diet and high in calories. I liked bread, pasta, rice, and cereals. I also started to count calories which I don't do any more.

A discussion with a dietitian on the way to the Chicago half-marathon also convinced me to eliminate all fat-reduced food and concentrate on whole, non-processed fresh foods. The dietitian's logic was that while the fat was reduced from the foods during processing, additional things like sugars and corn syrup were sometimes are added to improve the taste. Today Maria and I maintain a stable lean weight, follow no special diet but simply eat fresh, non-processed food which is typically low in carbohydrates but high in nutrition. It also includes plenty of fresh vegetables and fruit. I figured it's simple enough to follow and it works for us.

Eat right and light for a healthy heart. No one can beat a healthy heart.

Chapter 21

Marathons and other notable races

Rottnest Island — Australia	2004	
Perth — Australia	2005	with Maria
Rottnest Island — Australia	2005	with Maria
Singapore	2006	with Maria (plus 2007)
Hawaii — Big Island USA	2007	with Maria
Athens — Greece	2007	with Maria
Singapore	2008	with Maria
Sundown — Singapore	2008	with Maria
Great Wall — China	2008	with Maria
Egypt	2009	with Maria
Rio De Janeiro — Brazil	2009	with Maria

City to Surf Perth — Australia	2009	with Maria
Two Oceans — South Africa	2010	with Maria
City to Surf Perth — Australia	2010	with Maria
Singapore	2010	with Maria
Perth — Australia	2011	with Maria
Rottnest Island — Australia	2011	with Maria
City to Surf Perth — Australia	2011	
Antarctica	2012	with Maria
Perth — Australia	2012	
City to Surf Perth — Australia	2012	
Sydney — Australia	2012	with Maria
Rottnest Island — Australia	2012	with Maria
Los Angeles — USA	2013	with Maria
Seattle — USA	2013	with Maria
Pikes Peak Colorado — USA	2013	with Maria
Denver Colorado — USA	2013	
Montréal — Canada	2013	with Maria

Indian Creek Fifties Colorado — USA	2014	
Boston — USA	2015	with Maria

Notable half-marathons and other races

Chicago, USA	2013	with Maria
Cambodia — Angkor Wat, Cambodia	2009	with Maria
Georgetown, Colorado, USA	several	with Maria
Estes Park half-marathon, USA	2014	with Maria
Prairie Dog half-marathon — Denver USA	2015	
Perth, Australia	many	with Maria
SSAFRA half-marathon, Singapore	several	with Maria
Platte River half-marathon Denver, USA	several	with Maria
Singapore — 50 km duo race — first place	2010	with Maria
Fremantle, Perth, Australia	2005	with Maria
Singapore triathlons	several	with Maria
Perth, Australia triathlons	several	
Busselton 70.3 Ironman triathlon	2010	with Maria
Rocky Mountain Triathlon — highest triathlon in the world	2014	Marathon guide

Many of these races offer a great opportunity for first time marathoners. The ultramarathons and races like the Antarctic Marathon, Two Oceans Marathon, The

Great Wall Marathon, Indian Creek 50s and Pikes Peak Marathon would be less suitable for a first marathon experience but not impossible.

Rottnest Island Marathon, Western Australia, Australia
Key feature: Beautiful island location
Comment: Scenic location, relatively flat race, typically hot to very hot and dry, small number of participants, part of a running festival, involves four laps and is well-organised. The race is also an opportunity to stay and holiday on this beautiful pristine island off the coast of Western Australia. There was no race Expo.

Perth Marathon, Western Australia, Australia
Key feature: Flat, fast course
Comment: Nice location, relatively flat race along the Swan River, typically cool with reasonable number of participants. It's well-organised. The race is also an opportunity to visit Perth which is a beautiful city on the coast of Western Australia with sandy beaches and surf. There is no race Expo. This race offers an opportunity for a PB and a BQ

Singapore Marathon, Singapore
Key feature: Iconic run, well-organised and flat
Comment: Singapore is an interesting place to visit. Nice location, relatively flat race, typically hot and humid, large number of participants, part of a running

festival, involves a great route through the city, historic areas, East Coast and is well-organised. This would be good for first time marathoners. The race is also an opportunity to stay and holiday in this small but very interesting country. There was no significant Race Expo then.

Big Island Marathon, Hawaii, USA

Key feature: Scenic location

Comment: Relatively flat race along the coast, typically hot with a small number of participants. The race includes part of the Ironman marathon course. It's also an opportunity to stay and holiday in Hawaii. There was no race Expo then.

Athens Marathon, Greece

Key feature — Iconic, original marathon

Comment: Great opportunity to run from the town from which the marathon race takes its name. Follows a historic route to the marble stadium used for the first modern Olympics in Athens. The race is also an opportunity to stay and holiday in Athens and visit the famous Greek Islands. There was then no significant race Expo.

Sundown Marathon, Singapore

Key feature: Unusual race. Starts at midnight and offers an ultramarathon.

Comment: The route is along the East Coast of Singapore and it is well-organised. The race is a relatively flat race, typically hot and humid with a possibility of rain. The race is also an opportunity to stay and holiday in this small but very interesting country. There was no significant Race Expo then.

Great Wall Marathon, China

Key feature: Very challenging, adventure marathon in a unique historic location

Comment: This is a very demanding race and an opportunity see first-hand the Great Wall of China and run through some very interesting Chinese countryside. It can be hot, but the race is well-organised. This is not an opportunity for a PB or BQ. The race is also an opportunity to stay and holiday in China and visit famous cities like Beijing and Shanghai. There was no significant Race Expo then. When I did this race, I needed to enter using a specific travel company.

Egypt Marathon, Egypt

Key feature: flat, fast marathon in a unique, ancient, historic location.

Comment: Amazing historic location, relatively flat race, typically hot and dry with a smaller number of participants and supporters. It is part of a running festival and features a well-organised gala function in the evening. The race is also an opportunity to stay and holiday in this interesting country, visit the Valley of the Kings / Queens, the Pyramids, and their Ancient History museum. There was no race expo then.

Rio De Janeiro Marathon, Brazil
Key feature: relatively flat and spectacular coastline
Comment: This race offers an opportunity for a PB and a BQ and would be good for first time marathoners. Relatively flat race, typically hot, large number of participants, involves a start 42.2 kilometres (26.2 miles) to the north and a run along the coastline. It's well-organised. The race is also an opportunity to stay and holiday in Rio de Janeiro and Brazil.

City to Surf Marathon, Perth, Australia
Key feature: Flat, fast course with a few small hills, ends at a beautiful beach.
Comment: Nice race route, typically cool at the start and can warm up. Well-supported and part of a well-established running festival. The race is also an opportunity to stay and holiday in Perth and see the wonderful South West of this country. We both did a PB and BQ in this race.

Two Oceans Marathon, Cape Town, South Africa
Key feature: A very beautiful but challenging ultramarathon.
Comment: Scenic location, route involves steep inclines,

typically warm to hot, great supporters and well-organised. This is an iconic race in Cape Town. The race is also an opportunity to stay and holiday in Cape Town, visit Stellenbosch and visit a game park.

Antarctica Marathon, Antarctica

Key feature: Challenging, extreme marathon on a spectacular continent

Comment: People don't often get an opportunity to holiday in Antarctica, so this is a rare opportunity for marathoners plus tick Antarctica off your seven continents and holiday list. Can have extreme conditions like blizzards, very low temperatures, and unstable / icy footing. The race is well-organised together with a scenic boat cruise, small number of participants and opportunities for visiting penguin colonies and swimming / kayaking in Antarctica. It's not an opportunity for a PB or BQ.

Sydney Marathon, Sydney, New South Wales, Australia

Key feature: Relatively flat fast course in a spectacular harbour city.

Comment: Scenic location, typically cool to warm conditions, part of a running festival and is well-organised. I wasn't aware of a Race Expo then. The race is also an opportunity to stay and holiday in Sydney. It's a good race to do a personal best and a Boston Marathon qualifying time. I did both a PB and BQ.

Los Angeles Marathon, Los Angeles, California, USA
Key feature: Tour of LA, great spectators and ends at Santa Monica beach
Comment: I enjoyed starting at the Dodger Baseball Stadium. The race was relatively flat, well-organised, warm with many participants and great supporters. It had a very good race Expo. It's also a good opportunity to visit, stay and go to Disneyland, Hollywood Establishments like Warner Brothers and see the spectacular coastline.

Seattle Marathon, Seattle, Washington, USA
Key feature: Cool, well-supported undulating course
Comment: Scenic race route, undulating course, typically cool to warm in temperature. Large number of participants and has a half-marathon as well. There was a race Expo. The race is also an opportunity to stay and holiday is Seattle which is a beautiful coastal city.

Pikes Peak Marathon, Manitou Springs, Colorado, USA
Key feature: America's ultimate challenge — extreme marathon up to 14 000 feet
Comment: This is a very challenging race. It starts in Manitou Springs, Colorado USA and goes up to over 14 000 feet on trails to the top of the mountain and back again to the start. It's a trail race with, in many areas, poorly formed trails and significant rock obstacles. It has been rated as one of the toughest marathons in the world. There was no race Expo then.

Denver Marathon, Denver, Colorado, USA

Key feature: cool, fast, relatively flat marathon

Comment: Typically, cool but was cold when I ran. It's well-organised and well-supported with a good number of participants. There's a half-marathon as well. The race starts in the downtown area and ends there as well. There was a race Expo then. The race is also an opportunity to stay and visit Denver, Colorado, and the Rocky Mountains.

Montréal Marathon, Montréal, Quebec, Canada

Key feature: cool, fast marathon — good chance of a PB and BQ

Comment: Undulating race, typically cool with large number of participants and is well-organised. It's a good race to do a personal best and a Boston Marathon qualifying time. Maria and I both did BQ times in this race. Montréal is also a lovely place to visit.

Indian Creek Fifties Ultramarathon, Colorado, USA

Key feature: adventure ultra-trail marathon in spectacular wilderness

Comment: Trail ultramarathon with small number of participants and mountainous trails south of Denver in Colorado. There are two distances, 50 kilometres and 50 miles. The race is not an opportunity for a fast time but an opportunity to enjoy the pre-dawn start and the route through some spectacular Colorado mountain terrain. There was no race Expo. It's not that sort of event.

Boston Marathon, Boston, Massachusetts, USA

Key feature; Famous, since 1897, well-organised and well-supported

Comment: The race is the only regular marathon that required runners to have a qualifying time from a certified marathon. Runners are bussed out to a start and then run back to Boston. It's a relatively flat race but does have some hills. When we ran it was cold and wet but equally it can be hot and dry, so the weather is variable. There was a very good race Expo. Despite the cold wet weather supporters lined the entire race route. The race is also an opportunity to stay and holiday in historic Boston.

Epilogue

Jewel wrote that I encouraged her, when we were in Antarctica, to run more marathons and complete her Seven Continents quest. That's true. But she failed to mention that she encouraged us to meet in Dar es Salaam, Tanzania, East Africa, to drive across the country to Arusha and climb Mount Kilimanjaro, the highest free-standing mountain in the world. So, we all did that together. It's an extreme event as it is 5 895 metres (19 341 feet) above sea level at the top, but we enjoyed the adventure and camaraderie. The climb from the base camp up to the lip of the crater and along the crater edge to the apex is a very challenging thing to do. After Jewel departed, Maria, I, and our friend Cyndy cycled across Tanzania on mountain bikes through that wonderful countryside on trails and stayed in some basic country accommodation. We even stayed in a tent in Mkomazi National Park with lions and elephants roaming free. These are wonderful experiences in life and there are many more to come.

Maria spent several years on bone-strengthening medication and recently received the good news that her bone density has not only stabilised but strengthened slightly. So, what did she do then? She put her running shoes back on and started running the local Perry Lakes' 5-kilometre Park Run which turned into a weekly 10-kilometre (6-mile) bridges run in Perth, then a 14-kilometre (9-mile) run with our friend Sarah. Last weekend we mentioned to Sarah that perhaps she was ready for her first half-marathon. So, they searched and found the Sunset Coast half-marathon and booked themselves in, including our daughter Frances. Sarah is excited as it's her first half- marathon. Another candle has been lit! Maria reminded me of my own quote:

'What do runners do? Runners run! '
— Michael Le Page

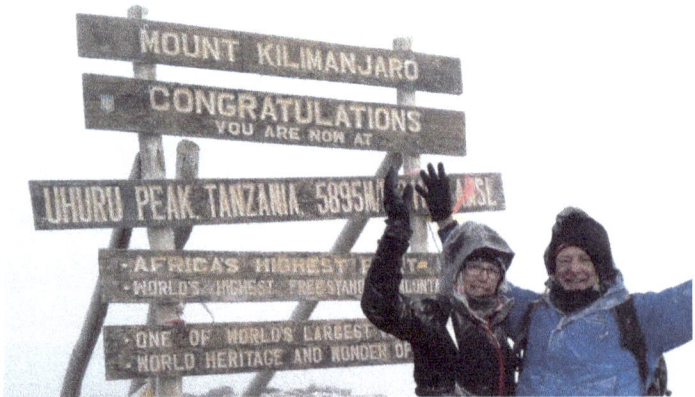

Photographs

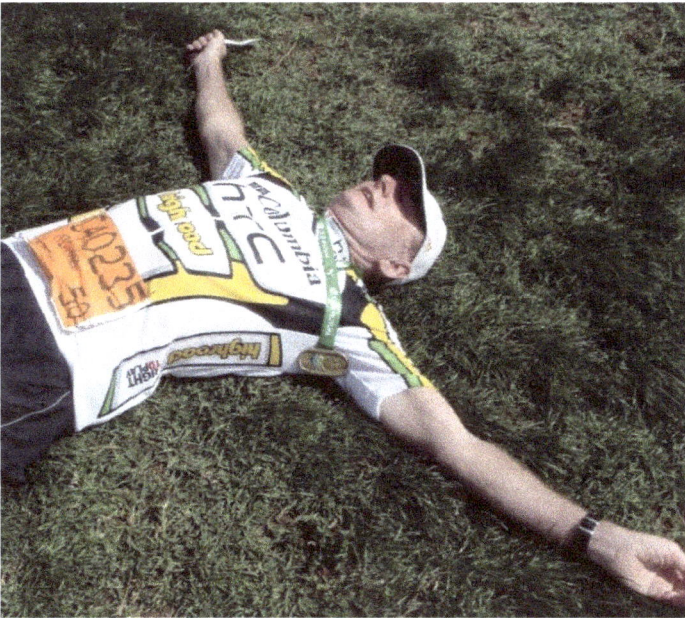

*Michael after finishing the Two Oceans ultramarathon in
Cape Town, South Africa*

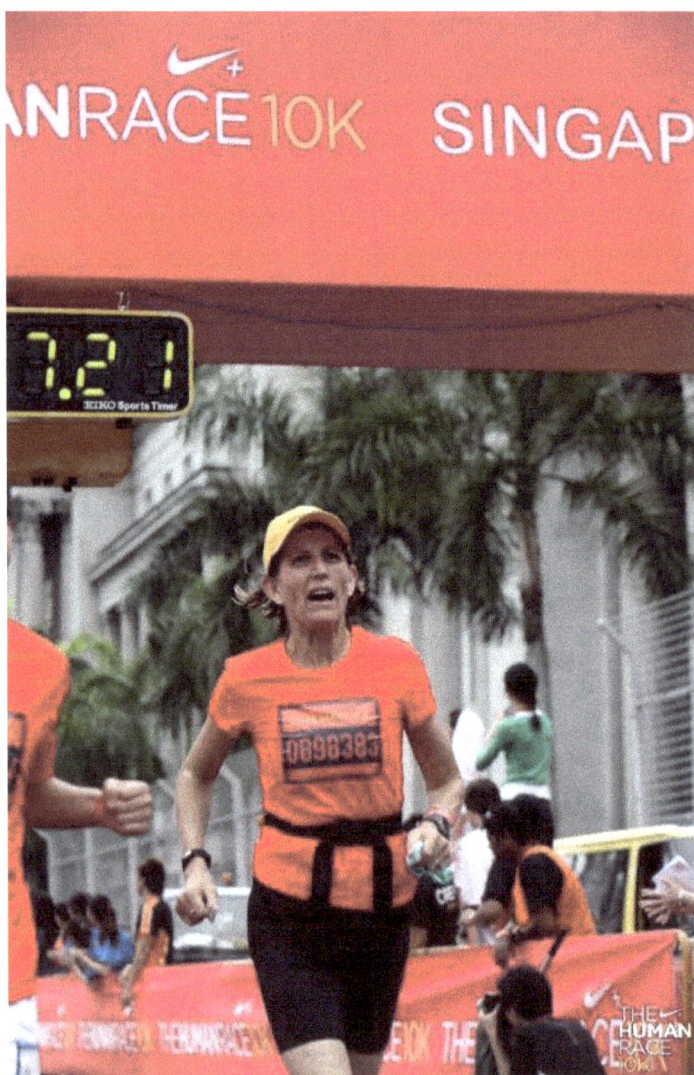

Maria — finishing a 10-kilometre race in Singapore

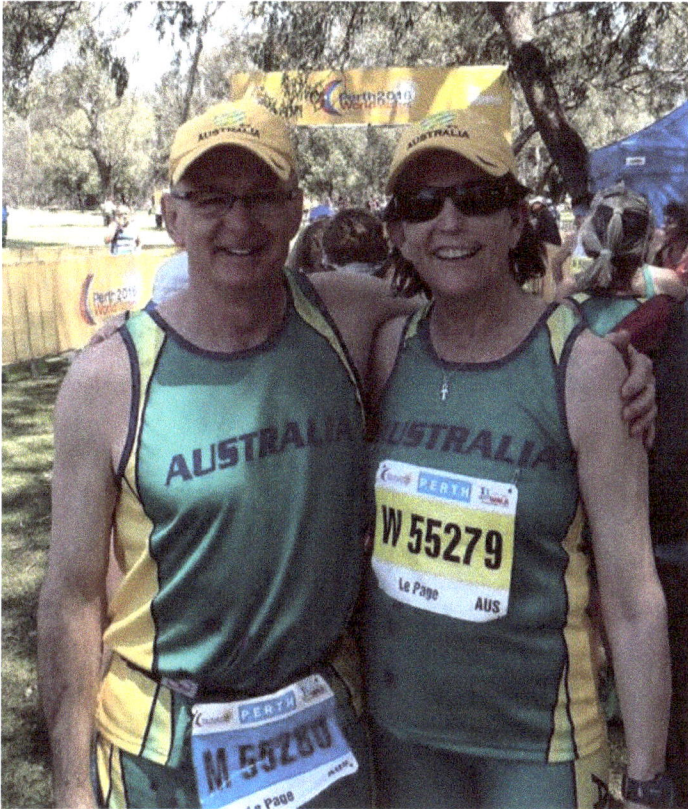

*Michael and Maria — Representing Australia
in the World Masters Athletics*

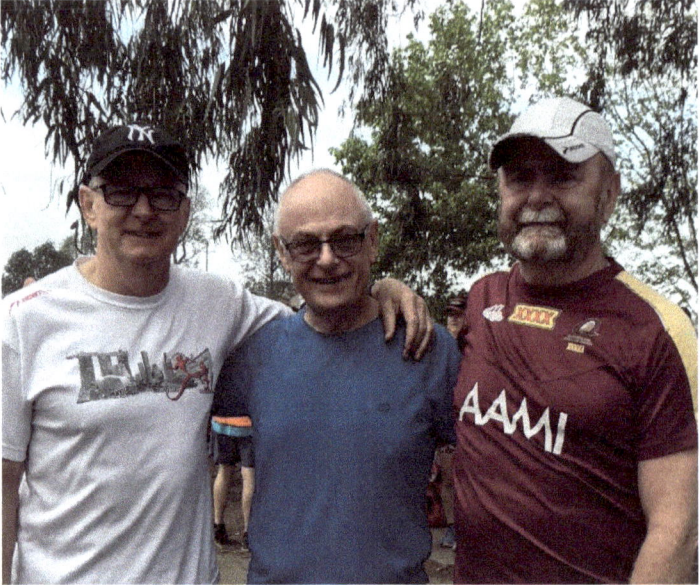

*Michael, my brothers John and Mark at a Park Run in
Maitland, Australia. Mark ran a marathon with me in Perth
and has run multiple half-marathons.*

John is in training for his first marathon.

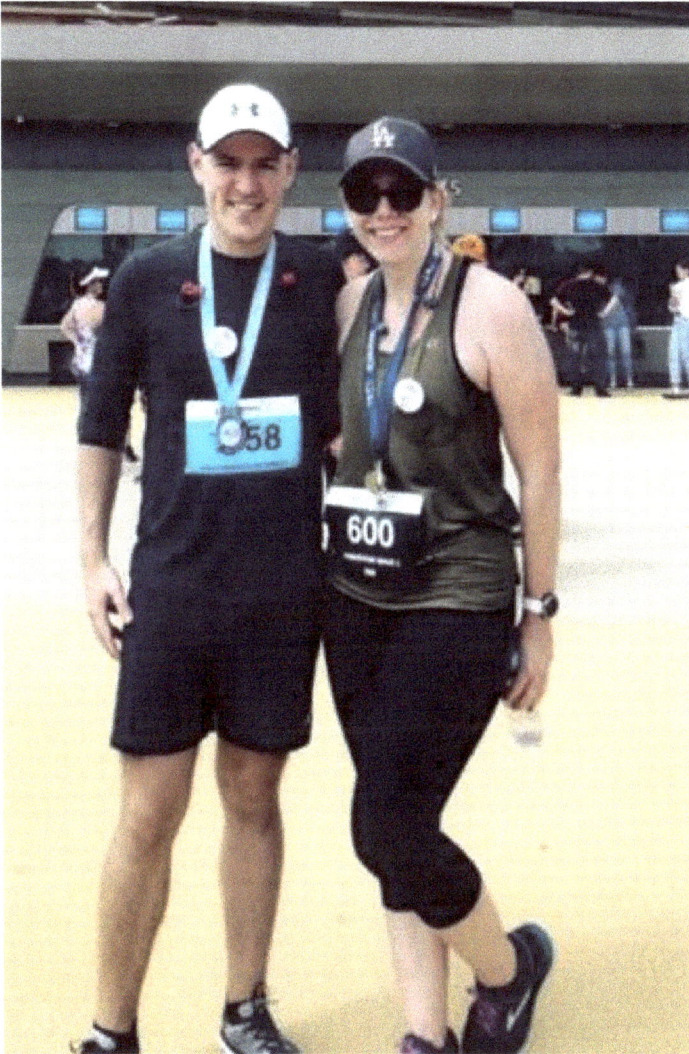

*Rob and Frances. Frances's first marathon
and Rob's half-marathon — Perth*

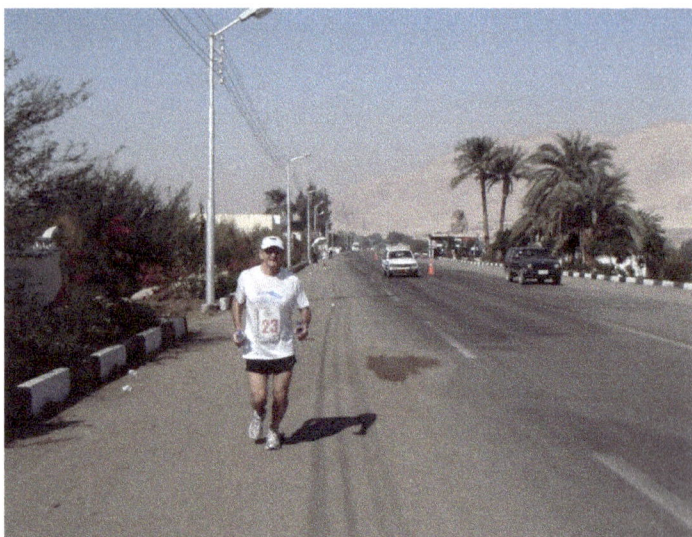

Michael — Egyptian marathon

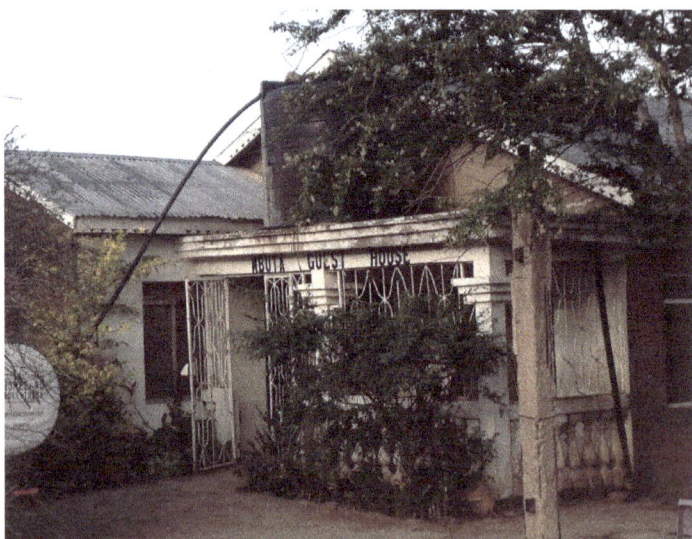

Accommodation in Tanzania

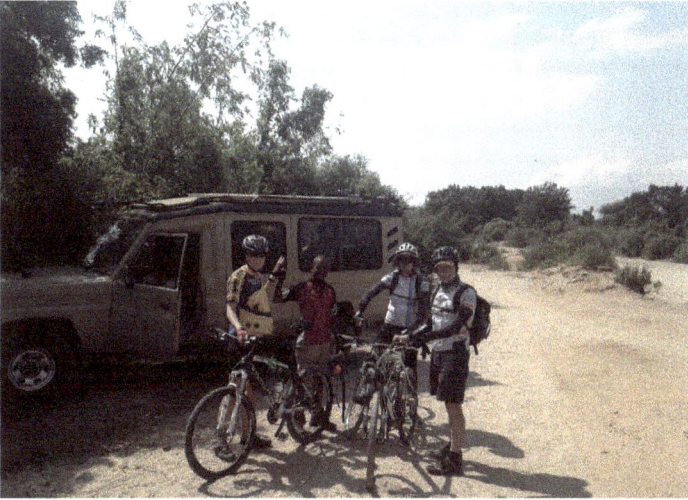

Cycling in Tanzania, East Africa

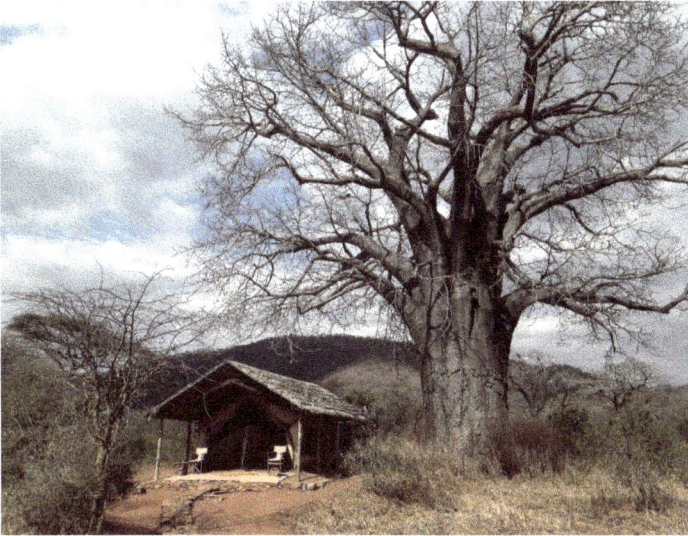

Tent in the national park — Tanzania, East Africa

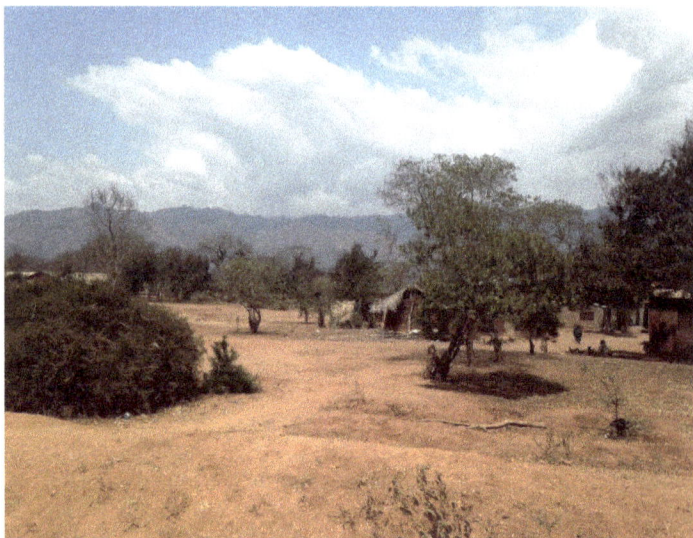

Tanzania — one of the villages we passed